# 8 Steps to Living a Long Life

"As a retired doctor of psychotherapy I am particularly interested in the psychological and physical impact this book will offer, ensuring good health and longevity. In addition to psychology, much of my professional career has been as a singer and singing teacher. The breathing techniques Peter teaches in this book are first-class for people who may suffer from a weakness in their breathing, typically caused by being physically blocked through poor deportment. These techniques will unlock, repair, and regulate the whole respiratory function. I suffer from osteoarthritis and myalgic encephalomyelitis (ME), an incurable chronic disease, and Peter's teachings have enabled me to function far more positively and productively than otherwise would have been possible.

In summary, I recommend this book for any age or state of health, as one that provides gentle and easy movements, very clearly explained, to maintain good health and a sense of well-being; to aid healing or to restore good health after illness; to improve living where full physical restoration may not be possible; or merely to work toward a long and healthy life."

— **CHRISTINE SIMONS,** M.D., DProf, DipPsych, Chartered Fellow CIPD

"Peter's new book makes us look at ourselves through a different lens— the lens of longevity. He emphasizes the importance of 'health now for longevity later,' and I believe all age groups and fitness levels will benefit from the sound work/life balance the Earth Path offers.

Elite sports would be wise to take notice of its guidance because super fit does not necessarily mean super healthy, and the truth is we all want to live long and die healthy. Having worked closely with Peter I know firsthand his knowledge and attention to detail, which shines through in this book."

— **TOM HEATON,** Manchester United and England International goalkeeper

# 8 Steps to Living a Long Life

## The Earth Path of Taoism

### Sifu Peter Newton

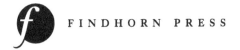

FINDHORN PRESS

Findhorn Press
One Park Street
Rochester, Vermont 05767
www.findhornpress.com

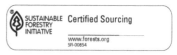

SUSTAINABLE FORESTRY INITIATIVE
Certified Sourcing
www.forests.org
SFI-00854

Text stock is SFI certified

Findhorn Press is a division of Inner Traditions International

**Disclaimer**
The information in this book is given in good faith and intended for
information only. Neither author nor publisher can be held liable by
any person for any loss or damage whatsoever which may arise from
the use of this book or any of the information therein.

Cataloging-in-Publication data for this title is available from the Library of Congress

ISBN 979-8-88850-140-5 (print)
ISBN 979-8-88850-141-2 (ebook)

Printed and bound in the United States by Lake Book Manufacturing, LLC.
The text stock is SFI certified. The Sustainable Forestry Initiative® program
promotes sustainable forest management.

10 9 8 7 6 5 4 3 2 1

Edited by Nicky Leach
Illustrations by Jeff Cushing and Peter Newton; see also Illustration Credits (p. 201)
Text design and layout by Anna-Kristina Larsson
This book was typeset in Garamond, Arida and Raleway

To send correspondence to the author of this book, mail a first-class letter
to the author c/o Inner Traditions • Bear & Company, One Park Street,
Rochester, VT 05767, USA and we will forward the communication,
or contact the author directly at **chinabridge_taichi@yahoo.co.uk**

The Chinese Art of Living is to be as healthy as one can, for as long as one can, and living as contented as one can.

~ Tong Sing, *The Chinese Book of Wisdom*[1]

# Contents

# Foreword

English psychoanalyst D.W. Winnicott, pondering the meaning of the word "culture," has this to say: "In any cultural field it is not possible to be original except on a basis of tradition."[2]

In his preface, Sifu Peter Newton tells us that the "insights, philosophy, and sources of knowledge" presented in his book are derived "from what the ancient masters discovered." This is evidenced in the knowledge he has distilled from his extensive reading of the Chinese classics and teachings of the historic figures of Taoism. The originality of this book lies in the capacity of its author to engage imaginatively with his material, a capacity to create a space for a questing mind open to the potential for ancient teaching and practices to have relevance and a practical application for us today in the West.

Sifu Peter's vision of a qigong that can benefit and impact people's health and well-being is inspirational for those of us privileged to be part of his teaching team. He is unique in seeing how the exercises he has developed and presents in this book can extend beyond the class setting into a complete qigong practice for everyday living.

In recent years, Sifu Peter has turned his focus toward the physical fitness of older people. While noting that "all age groups" will benefit from the exercises set out in the Eight Steps, the elderly are his particular concern. The prevention of falls is listed as one of the key benefits of tai chi, and the wonderful alternative road sign for old people (see page 44) wittily illustrates the passionate aim of this book: to offer people moving into older age the opportunity to benefit from the remedial and therapeutic techniques embedded in the qigong exercises.

A second readership the author addresses are those with health issues that impact their daily lives, people who are living with the debilitating effects of diseases such as Parkinson's. His work is a testament to Sifu Peter's ability to perceive how traditions belonging to two different worlds—Traditional Chinese Medicine and Western medical knowledge—can both, as Ted J. Kaptchuk notes, "affect and often heal human beings regardless of their cultural affiliation."[3]

A qigong master once asked why we learn qigong, these "healing arts," to which he gave his own answer: "I want to find out, is this hand really my hand? Is this leg really my leg?"[4] In the same way, Sifu Peter wants his readers to get to know how their bodies work. He uses the language of the body, its physiognomy, and its anatomical structures. Readers learn, for example, about the mechanics of breathing, with each step clearly set out with accompanying diagrams.

A number of features within the eight Earth Path steps help the reader find their way into the qigong exercises. Movement sequences, such as those shown in Step 8 of *Daoyin* 1 (The Hundred Arm Swings), are spelled out with a corresponding image. Particularly helpful are photographs of actual classes that bring the exercises to life and images that illustrate incorrect posture. These give readers a starting point from which to ease the body into adopting the correct posture (see Figure 10).

Informing and giving meaning to the qigong practices is the body's internal energy. Through his own deep connection to this life force, Sifu Peter leads us inward to an awareness of the flow of *qi* in the body, it is our guide along The Way of the Earth Path. Thus, *Nei Dan* (what is hidden: the inner-directed Yin of Earth), and *Wai Dan* (what is manifest: the outward-directed Yang of Heaven) are brought into harmony and balance in what Sifu Peter has called "total integrated body motion." The way to Heaven, our Sifu has so often told us in his classes, is through Earth. In this book, our feet are set firmly on the ground of qigong practice: the Earth Path.

**Mary Davies Turner, Ph.D.**
Poetry and Philosophy Tutor (Retired)
University of Wales Trinity St David, Swansea

# Preface

Greetings, everyone. Welcome to my latest book, which for me has been the most difficult to write, because it deals with a subject that has baffled the greatest brains on the planet for centuries: how to live long and die healthy?

In the Western world, we tend to occasionally live long and, in the main, die sickly. To die healthy after a long, fulfilled life is, to the ancient Chinese mind, the art of living. This principle not only weaves its way throughout the Far Eastern countries generally but was also found to a lesser degree in many of our Western ancient cultures.

> *Yang—life begins,*
> *Yin and Yang harmony—life fulfilled.*
> *Yin—life ends.*
>
> ~ Sifu

Like the ancient Chinese who sought the answers to the meaning of life, I have spent over 40 years pondering longevity and the creation of a healthy life. Motivated by the same hopes, fears, and aspirations we all have, the Chinese asked the same questions we ask, but they faced far tougher obstacles than we experience in our relatively mollycoddled modern times. Although my personal 68 years of life experiences certainly have enabled me to write this book, the majority of its insights, philosophy, and sources of knowledge derive from these discoveries by the ancient masters.

This book is not an academic exercise and is open and accessible to all. It reflects how I teach, through deciphering and translating the hidden gems of health and longevity. These gems are typically found (but much harder to decipher) in ancient Chinese literary classics, such as *I Ching (The Book of Changes), T'ai Shang Ch'ing-ching Ching (Cultivating Stillness), Tao Te Ching (The Book of the Way and Its Virtue), Huang Di Nei Ching (The Inner Cannon of the Yellow Emperor),* and *Chung-Li Ch'uan-Tao Chi (The Tao of Health, Longevity, and Immortality).*

The seed of the idea for this book was sown in 2007 after I experienced a life-changing neck injury—the result of a car accident in the late 1980s, but unbeknownst to me, I had been living with a small but significant cervical joint dislocation since that time. In 2017, this ticking time bomb exploded in class while I was demonstrating the application of Fajing, tai chi chuan's explosive power. Something clicked in my neck, and I knew it was serious.

Two specialists reviewed my case. After examining the results of my MRI scan, they told me that my condition was inoperable and my only option was to claim disability benefits as I was unlikely to be able to teach anymore.

Somewhat shocked, I reluctantly claimed and was awarded the benefit. However, just a few weeks into my newly enforced retirement life, I had a *shen* light bulb moment after another disturbed night's sleep, and the revelation was that I decided to solve this myself.

I had just spent 27 years learning the amazing remedial therapy techniques embedded in tai chi and qigong under the tutelage of three internationally revered grandmasters—Chu King-Hung, Michael Tse, and Dr. Yang, Jwing-Ming—and I believed that I could apply the techniques on myself.

After discussing my intentions with my wife, I decided to cancel my disability benefit and began an immediate staged comeback to the role I love: tai chi and qigong sifu. Gradually, over an 18-month period, I applied my Chinese therapy skills on myself and found the debilitating symptoms eased to the point that I could move virtually pain free. As I write, it is now 2023, and at the age of 68 I am moving with grace, balance, and flexibility and am robust in health.

This enlightening and, at times, taxing experience redirected my way of teaching and kick-started my research into ancient Chinese longevity and medical-based applications within the Taoist arts of tai chi and qigong. Consequently, I have spent the last 16 years guiding those who have lost their way to walk the Earth Path of Zhong-Li and Lu.

The Earth Path is the first of three major paths to health, longevity, and enlightenment described by two of the Eight Immortals of Chinese folklore: Zhong-Li Quan and Ancestor Lu Dongbin in their literary classic *Chung-Lu Ch'uan Tao Chi*. The Three Paths are Lesser (Earth), Middle (Heaven and Earth), and Greater (Heaven).

In the Introduction, I will explain how these paths can become a guiding focus that enables us to find ourselves when we feel lost. I also make reference to the Tao, Taoism, and their accompanying health, longevity, and spiritual enlightenment disciplines. I could not write a book on this subject without referring to the Fang Shih masters (Prescribers) who in ancient times were regarded as Taoist guides on all matters pertaining to spirituality, healing, and longevity. When taught and practised correctly, these three pillars of the Fang Shih will not only improve health and quality of life but can also extend its length.

In common with Fang Shih, every time I teach, where appropriate, I prescribe physical and psychologically beneficial remedies for conditions I note in others that they may not necessarily be aware of themselves. These beneficial remedies can mildly or dramatically improve the quality of life of an individual by clearing the physical and sometimes mental obstructions and blockages to the normal healthy flow of *qi*, the vital energy/life force that serves and sustains a healthy human body and mind.

In the pages that follow I will show you how to apply this information to yourself and others. It is information that I feel is vital guidance on your journey through life, where conflicting information is often furnished by myriad experts who not only contradict each other but sometimes themselves.

Chinese wisdom is consistent and still practised and promoted as it has been for thousands of years, because knowledge is timeless and what worked then has not aged or lost its effectiveness. There were periods in ancient Chinese history when living long and dying healthy was not just an aspiration; it was a normal transition. But even then, this was usually only for the adepts who chose to meticulously follow the teachings of the Taoist Earth Path. Now this path is open to you.

*The Tao is never far from humanity.*
*It is humanity that has moved away from the Tao.*[5]

~ Zhong-Li

This brings us to, who is this book for? The ideal readers of this book are teachers and practitioners of physical therapy, martial arts, tai chi, qigong, yoga, general health and fitness, and anyone with an interest in human longevity. This book will also, of course, be helpful for anyone living with chronic health issues that negatively impact their daily life and who may be feeling lost. Follow the guidance in this book, and you may discover that you have found yourself again. All age groups will benefit from this book; even younger children of eight and older can be gradually introduced to this material as they become mature enough to understand it.

So allow me to be your guide as you take your first exploratory steps along the first of the three paths. How far you go is up to you. My fervent hope that this book will help enlighten you so that you can find the balance that opens the door to a long, contented, and healthy life.

*Contemplate your navels,*
*Be as an open valley,*
*And soar like a crane.*

~ Sifu Peter Newton, November 2023

# Introduction

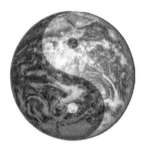

The eight Earth Path steps described in this book offer a unique opportunity to learn how the ancient Chinese realized their life-long ambition to live long and die healthy.

To help you physically learn and assimilate these steps, the book contains eight specially selected *daoyin* (guiding and leading) exercises that strengthen and rejuvenate the mind and body. The subtle combination of profound breathing supported by naturally aligned body structures and mechanics will guide your movements and lead healthy energy (*qi*) to all zones of the body. Robust health and a desire to lead an active, joyous life are the positive results—also in your golden years.

## Daoyin Origins

*Daoyin* is believed to be what the ancients called qigong, and its principles informed the formation of tai chi chuan, circa AD 1200. *Daoyin* can also be broken down as:

***Dao* = to guide the breath/*qi*:** The mind leads the *qi*, which is nourished by the breath.

***Yin* = to stretch the body:** Stretching the muscles, tendons, and ligaments of the whole body helps maintain the ROM (range of motion) in the joints and allows more space for the organs to breathe and function. In addition, stretching keeps the blood vessels and nerve fibres toned and youthful.

**Together, they bolster health for a long life.**

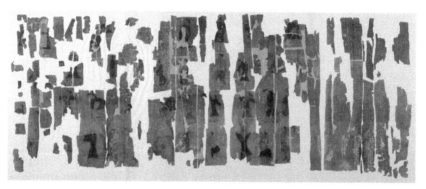

**Fig. 1** Original *Daoyin Tu* image from Han Dynasty

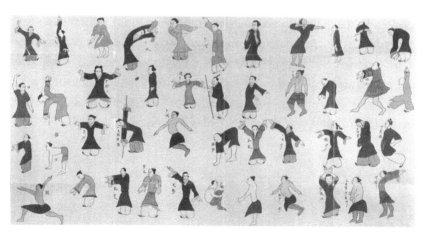

**Fig. 1a** Enhanced image of *Daoyin Tu*

The mottled and worn images depicted in Figure 1 were found in an unearthed tomb in Mawangdui, Hunan Province by Chinese archaeologists in 1973. In the enhanced image shown in Figure 1a, you can fully appreciate the range and sophistication of the *daoyin* depicted, especially considering that this was over 2,000 years ago. It shows images of people during the Han Dynasty (circa 168 BC) performing *daoyin* exercises painted onto silk and is entitled *The Daoyin Tu*.

All eight *daoyin* longevity exercises in Step 8 have their roots in these ancient images and remain true to the originals. Only seasoned professionals who have mastered a wide range of Chinese exercises will recognize most of the images depicted in *The Daoyin Tu*, and it is surprising how many have survived to this day.

Of course, the illustrations depicted here are only a snapshot of the range of *daoyin* that would have existed, and it is sad to ponder how many have been lost in the mists of time. Following all of the steps chronologically, from 1 to 8 (and even beyond), will offer remedial therapy for a variety of common human health conditions and unlock your potential.

## Tao and the Three Paths

Taoism forms the greatest influence in this book and, therefore, it is wise at this juncture to put the Tao and its belief system, Taoism, on the map. *Tao* literally means "The Way," which is the origin of all things in the universe and the destructive and creative forces that we see in everything, including ourselves.

It is not a conventional religion, as in its simplest form its adepts (Taoists) are followers of The Way, with no deity, just majestic nature and its impact on our lives at its heart. Unlike Buddhism, with its belief system based on the teachings of the Buddha, Taoism has more than one iconic figure at its centre. Those with the greatest notoriety are Lao Tzu, Chuang Tzu, Ko Hung, Shou Lao, Zhong-Li Quan, and Lu Dongbin (Ancestor Lu). It is the latter two who bring the three paths to our attention.

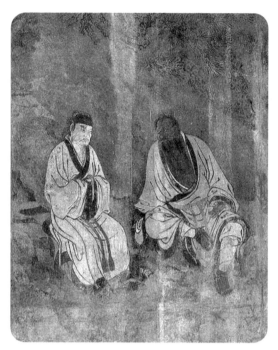

**Fig. 2** 14th-century painting of
Zhong-Li Quan instructing Lu Dongbin

Zhong-Li and Lu are regarded as two of the most recognizable characters in Taoist history. Their literary classic *The Tao of Health and Longevity* records the dialogue held between teacher Zhong-Li and pupil Lu, despite both apparently existing in different dynastic periods: Zhong-Li (Han Dynasty, 206 BC–AD 226) and Lu (Tang Dynasty, AD 618–906).

Another notable literary gem, which should only be consulted when following the Middle and Greater Paths, is *The Secret of the Golden Flower*, a Taoist-based book on inner essence cultivation (*neidan*) through meditative practice and immortality guidance notations. It is said to have been written by Lu Dongbin and/or disciples of the Complete Reality School, a school founded by Lu, which fused Taoist, Buddhist, and Confucian teachings. In addition, Lu is famous as the scribe of the *Bai Zi Bei* (The Hundred Character Tablet), an historic discourse offering guidance on how to attain immortality in one hundred characters.

# Philosophical *Koans*

To help understand their philosophy of life and the universe, each of the eight steps in the book features *koans*: typical philosophical conversations that may have occurred between student Lu (presumably at the start of his journey on the path to enlightenment) and the wise, enlightened master Zhong-Li. Here is an example of such a koan:

## Zhong-Li and Lu Discuss Searching for the Tao

**Lu:** Master, we have travelled many miles this day, and yet you seem to be less tired than myself. Why is this?

**Zhong-Li:** My steps are lighter than yours, and my body may look heavy but is lighter than yours.

**Lu:** But how is it possible? I am slimmer and lighter in frame and even younger than you.

**Zhong-Li:** You still carry the weight of the world throughout your body, and the Tao is as yet not walking with you. Whereas I am open as a valley, and I soar and breathe like a crane–vitality seeks me, whilst you seek it.

**Lu:** Are you saying my mind has not caught up with us here in our mountain retreat, because it still carries the stresses of human life and therefore makes my body heavy with the same stresses?

**Zhong-Li:** The Tao mind is clear as a mountain stream, whereas yours remains cloudy. It is time for you to embrace the Now and release the bondages of your past.

**Lu:** Master, I have also noticed that we tread on virgin ground. No path lies before us, and yet you stride out as if you have a clear destination. Where are we going?

**Zhong-Li:** When I walked amongst humans, *they* determined the paths I should follow. Whereas here, all paths lead to the Tao; we are already at our destination.

*The Tao of Health, Longevity, and Immortality* referred to above is written for Taoist teachers and adepts to decipher, interpret, and transmit its contents to enlighten future generations. The scripture is full of incredible insights into how to attain sustained health and longevity and if inspired enough, to pursue the ultimate goal: *tai shang* (immortality).

According to Zhong-Li and Lu there are three stage paths to health, longevity, and enlightenment for us mere mortals:

1 **The Lesser (Earth) Path:** This path is the theme for this book. As described by Immortal Zhong-Li, it is the path whereby mortal humans are able to "cultivate a strong body that is immune to many diseases, allowing them to enjoy good health and live a long life in the human realm." It is for people who walk the earth and are susceptible to human weaknesses (mental and physical) and searching for a way to rectify their unsatisfactory lives.

2 **The Middle (Heaven and Earth) Path:** According to Zhong-Li, this path is "concerned with the cultivation of extended longevity (along a strong, centred life-line)." It is for people who have overcome human weakness and are ready to walk the Middle Path to an extended healthy life.

3 **Greater (Heaven) Path:** This path is described as being "concerned with the cultivation of Immortality." It is for Lohans; that is, people whose state of health and expansion of mind has evolved to such an extent they are ready to enter the gate of immortal training.

The three paths serve as stepping stones to a higher state of being. Even in those days, they were sequentially attempted by very few people, or even the chosen few. Today, nothing has changed. People attempting the enlightenment journey are a select few, a situation that is unlikely to alter in the foreseeable future.

In this book, I hope to inspire more of us to take the first tentative steps towards Earth Path enlightenment, because the Lesser Earth Path was always intended for the masses due to its simple and achievable message.

The exact content of the Earth Path curriculum is not clear; however, this book will attempt to pull all the clues together to produce as close as possible what the enlightened sages would have proposed:

MIND—BODY—SPIRIT—HEAVEN—EARTH—

HUMAN—YIN—YANG—REJUVENATION—

ALTERATION—ILLUMINATION

All the life-changing aspects above are covered in the pages of this book and placed in specific sequence to guide the recipient gently and carefully along the Lesser (Earth) Path of health, healing, and longevity.

Those who complete the transition offered by the Lesser (Earth) Path described in this book will find it much easier to navigate the Middle (Heaven and Earth) Path of Longevity. The Middle Path is designed to teach you how to centre the mind, body, and spirit, creating a condition in the physical body called "central equilibrium," in which the physical human form becomes perfectly balanced between Heaven and Earth. The ancient Chinese also called this stage of evolutionary development *San Tsai*, meaning "Three Powers," where the mind, body, and spirit are united with the interactive powers between Heaven and Earth.

Central equilibrium was initially taught while on the Lesser Path and developed further on the Middle Path. Internally, it leads to the *jing lo* ("energy meridian body") being switched on. The aim of this stage is to lead the individual to the hallowed entrance of the Greater Path and extend the Earth Path beyond what is normally expected (a life span of 100 years should be regarded as a mere stepping stone).

The third stage is called the Greater Path of Heaven and leads Lohans—those who are ready—to spiritual awakening and enlightenment. To date, writings fail to clarify what this enigmatic aspiration entails; it is normally presented in bafflingly cryptic form. However, it is fair to say that this level of awakening is unlikely to be achieved without completion of the two previous paths, and anyway, those who have returned home to the Tao (as it is called) do not advertise the fact and would deny it if pressed.

# Preview of the Eight Steps

### Step 1
## Illumination of *Yangsheng*

This step introduces the Earth Path and why this path is intended for those who, according to the Tao mind, are lost. Lost people need guidance, grounding, and rooting. These themes are addressed sequentially throughout the book, but Step 1 explains how people get lost in the first place and identifies the root cause, be it self-imposed or accidental. The activated Earth Path switches on what the Chinese call *yangsheng* ("nourishing life") and steers us towards a healthy, long, and contented life. The book explores different scenarios, cross-referenced to the relevant steps, with the intention of helping avoid future mistakes in life or remedying those already made.

### Step 2
## *Zhang Luanli*—The Long Principle

This step explains how to apply the Chinese concept of *zhang* ("long") into all areas of your life. This brings us firmly onto the Earth Path, as every journey starts with the first step. During the decades I have studied under the masters, all have regularly used the word "long" in their references; for example: "Breathe long, so that the *qi* will sink into your energy centre (located in the lower abdomen)." They, along with the ancients, also refer to other applications of where and when to apply the Long Principle, and Step 2 visits them all.

## Step 3
### *Shen Huxi*—Profound Breathing

This step focuses on transforming the biorhythm of unhealthy, shallow mouth breathing to one of healthy, deep, nasal breathing. It interprets the breathing guidance of enlightened beings from a bygone age and reveals its profound nature, drawing comparisons between modern health science recommendations and the old Taoist Masters.

## Step 4
### Secrets of the Longevity Icons

This step looks at real and mythical icons of longevity who reputedly lived to over 100 years of age, and examines their recommendations in order to inspire you to walk the Earth Path with vigour and emulate their achievements.

## Step 5
### *Yin* and *Yang* Rhythms of Life

This step teaches you how to attune to the natural circadian bio-rhythms needed for this journey. It compares a life out of step with the Tao with one lived in harmony with it, and includes a Yin and Yang lifestyle chart that illustrates how to bring this essential harmony into your life.

## Step 6
### *Jing Zuo*—How to Sit Quietly

This step shows the correct way to gaze inwards and discover the still-ness within. Stillness creates the perfect atmosphere to strengthen the mind, body, and spirit for the successful completion of the Earth Path and encourages beneficial changes to the body's sophisticated chemistry that are needed to help fight disease (disease is when a body is no longer "at ease"). The step includes do's and don'ts of *jing zuo* to ensure it is practised in the correct and natural way.

## Step 7
## Stirring the Shen—The Hidden Taoist Secret

This step offers a first look at engaging the *shen*, the inner potential of the human psyche, integral to Middle Path training, using illustrations and quotations from the Taoist Masters to shine a light on this jewel of practice. *Shen* is the ultimate motivator for improving health and vitality. The simple foundation techniques offer immediate benefits especially for those with low self-esteem and motivation.

## Step 8
## Eight *Daoyin* Longevity Exercises

This final step lays out eight *daoyin* longevity exercises, using words and photos to ensure they are practised correctly and safely. Descriptions include information on the health-enhancing benefits and why these exercises are key to the completion of the Earth stage of the longevity journey, as each one targets and rejuvenates key zones of the body while embracing the mind. The movements can be performed by all ages, seated or standing.

These collective actions create what the ancient Chinese referred to as the "Eight-Strand Brocade" of health, which cannot be torn and is essential to longevity. Each strand is a therapeutic physical exercise, which practised on their own, offer limited benefits; however, when combined, the eight selective therapeutic and complimentary exercises create a strong "brocade" with potentially unlimited benefits. In China, the number eight is regarded as special because it represents infinity, balance, power, strength, wealth, and good fortune.

## Ask Sifu: Q & A on Life and Longevity

This final section covers questions typically asked by inquisitive students and the author's response. The intention is to bridge any gaps in the information provided and allow you to follow the Earth Path with all the necessary information in hand.

In summary, *qi* (life-force energy) lies at the heart of this book, and the Eight Steps are designed to open the body and allow its streams and rivers to flow, unblocking trapped, negative, sickly *qi*. You will learn how to sense and feel *qi* ebbing and flowing along the *meridians* (energy channels of the body) and harness it. You could say this book provides *feng shui* for life.

> *Blockage creates stagnation.*
> *It's stagnation that ultimately kills you.*
> ~ Traditional Chinese Medicine maxim

## Roots of the *Fang Shih*

The knowledge and methods contained in the Eight Steps were certainly influenced and, some say, crystallized by the practices of the ancient Chinese Taoist physicians known as the Fang Shih and the generations of tai chi chuan and qigong masters who followed.

The Fang Shih (see Figure 3 below) were practising physicians, prescribers, shamans, diviners, alchemists, and mediums who can be traced back to a period between the 2nd century BC and the 4th century AD. The late John Blofeld, expert and author on ancient Taoism, makes the case for mentioning the Fang Shih when discussing the roots of health and longevity wisdom, writing in *Taoism and Quest for Immortality*: "The ancient Chinese Fang Shih masters achieved fame as physicians and were able to retain youthful vigour and live long."

These earliest recorded forerunners of what we recognize today as Taoist priests (*dao shih*) are believed to have been the evolutionary descendants of the Yin and Yang school of philosophy (circa the

3rd century BC). It is highly likely, therefore, that the roots of *feng shui* ("wind and water geomancy") lie within the practices of the Fang Shi. Feng shui masters are known for their skill in guiding people to maintain balance between Yin and Yang. The basis of their knowledge was likely informed by a cosmological view of the Heavens (Yang in nature) and Earth (Yin in nature) with all their prolific and profound interactions. The Fang Shih formed the bedrock on which Traditional Chinese Medicine (TCM) was built, it is believed, and would likely have prescribed similar exercises to the eight *daoyin* exercises laid out in Step 8.

*Taoist individualists* (Fang Shih) *who were looked upon with awe and reverence, would participate in society and even in government, offering an extra dimension of insight to bear on the problems of the time.*[6]

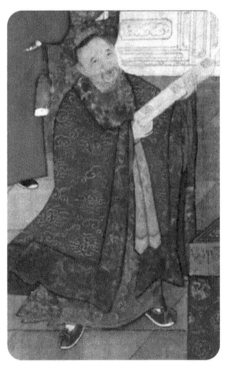

**Fig. 3** Shao Yuan Je, Zhengyi Dao's Taoist priest to the Jiajing emperor of the mid-Ming Dynasty. Dao Shih *(Fang Shih)*

The Fang Shih would mediate between human and spiritual realms, meaning that they would activate their "sky eyes" (the third eye located between the eyebrows mid-forehead, or *yin tang* in Chinese) and "heaven's gateway" (Hundred Convergences Crown Point located on the crown of the head, *baihui* in Chinese) to support their diagnosis and prognosis by reading their patients whilst drawing guidance from their celestial guides. Using their accumulated wisdom, Fang Shih masters would prescribe remedial actions that would no doubt have also included herbal and dietary remedies, both of which are outside of the scope of this book.

So what was it about the Fang Shih that was so attractive to the public and leaders, such as Emperor Han Wu-ti (140–87 BC)? One interesting observation of Chinese traditional belief that has travelled through the mists of time states, "How can an unhealthy physician heal me when they are unhealthy?" This corresponds with the earlier description in John Blofeld's book that the Fang Shih could "retain their youthful vigour and live long."

One term widely used in Chinese martial arts can be traced back to the time of the Fang Shih: *kung fu*, which, basically translated, means "time, patience, plus disciplined practice." In order to develop their fabled youthful health and vigour and live long, the Fang Shih would have needed nothing less than *kung fu*, and it is in the spirit of *kung fu* that you should apply yourselves to achieve your own goals.

# Tai Chi Chuan and Qigong

It is generally believed that the original *daoyin* system of exercising, with over 7,000 years of history, has been absorbed into the fabric of tai chi and qigong; therefore, it is important to briefly introduce these health and martial arts to you.

## Tai Chi Chuan

*Tai chi chuan* translates to "grand ultimate fist boxing" and was plainly intended to be a martial art. Reputedly, it has its origins in the 13th century AD and is attributed to a gentleman by the name of Chang San Feng (See Figure 31) who, on Wudang Mountain in Hubei Province, was thought to have created the first stages of tai chi chuan.

Interestingly, the idea for tai chi came to Chang San Feng after he witnessed a white crane fighting a snake—the coiling and evasiveness of the snake was matched by the lightness of footwork and lightning strikes of the crane. The crane has gone on to be more represented in tai chi postures than any other creature; other creatures featured include the sparrow, snake, monkey, tiger, cockerel/pheasant, and horse, all of which contribute their *teh* (character) to the spirit of the exercise/martial art system.

Tai chi's notoriety derives from its unique and subtle blend of posture engineering, body mechanics, coordinated breathing, and mind-focusing techniques, which create perfection in motion for the practitioner. It is constructed from a montage of martial art postures that are stitched together like a string of pearls to make what is known as a "form."

It is the "form" that is known worldwide for its grace and beauty, making the tai chi practitioner look like they are moving through water, and it is the "swimming in air" slow motion driven by mind-intent and deep, centreline, relaxed ("long") breathing that creates its great health benefits. The natural yet sophisticated movements embody the dynamics of Yin and Yang.

### Yang

Stretching upwards and outwards (expansion), linked to inhalation, which drives the soft tissue expansion (organs, nerve fibres, muscles, tendons, ligaments, connective tissue, blood vessels, lymphatic vessels, and skin tissue). All receive an influx of oxygen-enriched blood and, according to Chinese medicine, organs and their supportive tissues are encouraged to breathe, as is the whole body (*ti huxi*).

## Yin

Recoiling downwards and inwards (contraction), linked to exhalation, which returns the whole body to its natural repose and involves all the soft tissues referred to above shrinking back and emptying, which cleanses the body of toxins.

## Gravitational Yin and Yang

The gravitational forces acting upon the human frame when at rest and standing in a neutral Stand Long posture (See Figure 8) spread the load equally throughout the structural frame (Yin and Yang combine in stillness). This is a body at ease and in natural repose; however, as soon as movement in the form of weight transference is activated, gravitational force plus body mass condense down a single leg, creating what the ancient masters call Solid/Full Footing.

The leg that is now carrying the body mass is loaded further by gravitational force and becomes the single, solid root of the body. This results in firing up the structural bone's piezoelectric charge resulting in healthier bone cells and marrow (Yin is now dominant, separate from Yang yet still mutually connected). In this phase, you experience a dual sense of grounding and rooting and develop a profound feeling of stability.

As the body transitions to move the weight across to the opposite leg, an anti-gravitational upward force is generated making the once solid leg now hollow and empty (Yang is now dominant separated from Yin and also still mutually connected). In this phase you experience a sense of lightness bordering weightlessness, developing a profound feeling of freedom of movement.

## Tai Chi Circles

Traditionally, there exist three distinct circles (spheres of operation) in Yin and Yang motion within the art of tai chi (it exists in qigong also): small, medium, and large. Beginners would naturally gravitate to the large circle, while the intermediate and advanced would settle on medium and small circles, respectively:

**Large:** expansive, open, stretching, high stance, peripheral body focussed and the realm of those with limited range of movement in their joints.

**Medium:** centred, balanced, natural range of motion, a middle height stance and operating motion, spread evenly throughout the whole body.

**Small:** condensed, globally spiralling (although it can be localised— zoned in one area of the body) and the home of the masters.

It is interesting to note that along the journey to become a master of tai chi and qigong, the three circles have to be worked through in their natural order: large, medium, small. However, upon reaching the small and most advanced stage, you realize that you have to consistently embrace the other two circles otherwise you would stiffen up and lose your above average range of movement in your joints. The reason this is highlighted is because all three have their place in tai chi, qigong/*daoyin* exercise, and beyond this book, it is wise to seek a teacher who can demonstrate these circles of motion.

## The *Tai Chi* Symbol

The tai chi symbol is called *tai chi tu* (see Figure 4). It depicts these two most powerful forces in the universe harmonized into a perpetual cosmic dance in perfect balance. Through this balance all things are created and destroyed in a cosmic cycle of life and death.

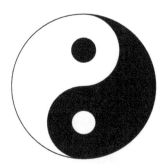

**Fig. 4** *Tai chi tu*

## *Tai Chi* Form

In Figure 5, you can see how a large group of people can also operate in mutual harmony when practising tai chi form. Each individual mirrors the next, and through this choreographed meshing you become one of the energy ripples of the collective. The fusing of minds and bodies creates an almost psychic sense of togetherness unseen in any Western style exercising. The "form" typically can be made up of 24, 37, or 108 postures, and each posture is engineered to human perfection in stillness and motion.

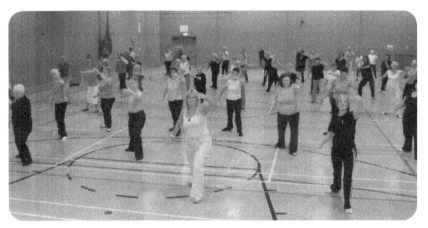

**Fig. 5** Charity event group practising *tai chi* form

In addition, the interaction of these body mechanics coupled with deep, relaxed, "long" breathing creates harmony between the internal and external. "Internal" refers to the energy circuitry (*qi jinglo*), breathing (*huxi*), and mind intent (*yi*), while "external" refers to the physical body, skin, muscles, and visible expressed power. When both are in harmony, Yin and Yang dance a ballet of such grace and mutual support they create perfection in physical balance, health, and general life.

## Health Benefits of Tai Chi

- Regulates posture to allow an even spread of gravitational force and motion
- Coordinates the body to create total integrated body motion (TIBM)

- Creates perfection in body mechanics
- Generates natural enhanced physical strength
- Trains the body to return to healthy "long" breathing
- Integrates breathing with body motion
- Regulates blood pressure by ironing out the kinks and creases in our bodies
- Raises the spirit of vitality by introducing you to your *shen*
- Centres and calms the mind, helping those with mental health issues
- Is the ultimate representation of what Lao-tzu called "methodical calmness"
- Swimming in air directly stimulates the mind and body's connection with space.

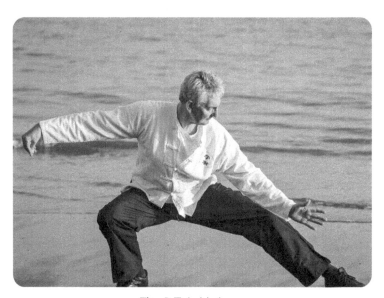

**Fig. 6** *Tai chi chuan*

## Medical Tai Chi

Even though it goes by this title, its full title is "medical tai chi chuan and qigong." This particular branch of tai chi is gaining momentum in the Western world, especially in hospitals, due to it dove-tailing comfortably with Western medical methodology. It combines the best of tai chi and qigong, and focuses on adapting their body mechanics, specially selected exercises, and therapeutic breathing routines.

Supplementary to this is the application of *an mo qigong* (combined massage and physical qigong exercise), *pai da* (tapping and slapping therapy), and *yaojing gong* (shaking therapy). In conjunction with the mindset of *jing zuo* and the inner sensing/gazing of *nei gong*, the methods are proving to be a potent force in clearing stagnation, while naturally regulating the whole body.

In this style of teaching, we come across *qu huxi* ("zone breathing"), which is when a specific zone of the body is manipulated through massage and concentrated physical movement, while focusing the breathing into the zone ("condensing breathing," or *leng ning huxi*). This is an excellent way to clear blockages caused by poor posture, adhesions, or mechanical damage. By combining the above, the normally stagnant stiff tissues are softened and released, and therefore, able to breathe and circulate once more.

# Qigong

Qigong is mainly practised for medical, health, and wellbeing reasons, so it can be applied for general health maintenance or targeted health issues. As mentioned earlier, in its early life it was generally known as *daoyin gong* ("training to guide and lead life-enhancing *qi*"). As previously noted, qigong ("energy training") is considered to be 7,000 years old, even though it identified as *daoyin* originally. The postures demonstrated in Step 8 are qigong/*daoyin* but also contain the postural excellence, mechanics, and mind-focusing techniques of tai chi chuan.

Step 8 will guide and lead you to perform the routines in a way to suit your experience level, so you should not feel overawed by the challenge ahead. Qigong can be performed standing or sitting, stepping or still; each has their place, making it much easier for people with limited mobility to enjoy the benefits. It is generally designed to work with the body in a manner that totally harmonizes with its natural rhythms. Like tai chi, qigong encourages both the moving and still body to operate in line with gravitational force, and as such, eliminates unnecessary wear and tear, especially on the joints. Perfection of movement, combined with "long," profound breathing and a stilled mind, switches a system of general exercise (external) to a total integrated mind/body discipline (internal and external).

## Health Benefits of *Qigong*

- Naturally tones and stretches muscles and tendons
- Loosens joints and ligaments
- Increases the body's general flexibility
- Stimulates the efficient function of organs and the endocrine system
- Blood and intercellular fluids are oxygenated
- The body becomes more alkalized rather than carbon-linked acidified
- Calms the central nervous system
- Trains how to store and regulate the life-force *qi*
- Targets specific organs remedially
- Places gravity at the centre of the joints
- Helps to slow biological ageing.

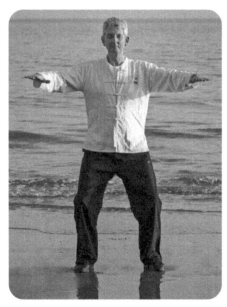

**Fig. 7** *Zhan Ma Bu Qigong,* (Standing Horse Stance training)

# Conclusion

Hopefully, this introduction will have clarified the origins of the Eight Steps and helped you appreciate the great depth of knowledge and wisdom contained within these sources. We are blessed in these times to not only benefit from the wisdom of the ancients but the accumulated tried-and-tested wisdom since those enlightened times.

"The answer you seek is within you, but it may be hard to find," Confucius is believed to have said. His comment illustrates how difficult it would have been to become enlightened (typically via the Earth Path) over 2,000 years ago, in an age with no "information highway" and a time when the knowledge was still in its embryonic stage of development.

Now, however, you can access this life-changing wisdom, and who knows how far you potentially could travel along the paths of Zhong-Li and Ancestor Lu?

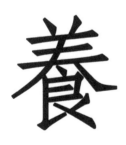

*Yang*—Nourish

*Sheng*—Life

# Step 1
# Illumination of Yangsheng

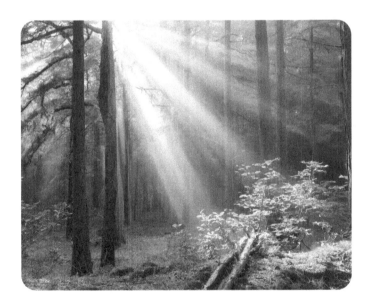

Lao Tzu the great Taoist mythical philosopher sage once said, "A journey of a thousand miles begins with the first step." This is where that step must be taken upon the Earth Path of Zhong-Li and Lu, and a most enlightening experience it is, too.

Some people stride along this pathway of life and achieve the ultimate goal: to live to a ripe old age and remain contented and healthy throughout. Others may not be so fortunate and find ill health has come to visit, either from birth or arrives later in life. Its impact is not only felt personally but it ripples out and negatively affects their closest family and friends. It destroys dreams and aspirations, lowers self-esteem and confidence, and causes stress and anxiety, introducing more conditions that compound the existing problem.

As you stumble along the Earth Path, not knowing what lies before you, this is where you will discover that there is another way. It is time to sit quietly (*jing zuo*) and look back at yourself with fresh unemotional eyes, as if you are assessing someone else. If you are living with or without health conditions, be they mental or physical, you can learn from what is about to unfold.

# Yangsheng

*Yangsheng* ("illumination") is a sensible first step along the Earth Path, as it is concerned with nourishing life, promoting vitality and health, and living long. It should start at an early age and remain throughout life, but for those just now stepping into the light after perhaps having spent most of their life in darkness, it is better late than never.

The term *yangsheng* breaks down as follows:

*Yang*—**Nourish:** This is where you embrace life and live it to the full, while maintaining the protection of the Yin and Yang Cycle of Life (See Figure 33) and conducting your life with a consistency centred on self-preservation. The word nourish has a broad meaning, including to feed, sustain, nurture, and cultivate. "But we do that anyway," I hear you say, and you would be right. But can you honestly say that you are doing the best for yourself? No doubt your intentions are pure and sincere, but you may be falling just short of the desired level of nourishment necessary.

*Sheng*—**Life:** This refers to life in its purest sense—present in the newborn baby, the earliest shoots of life itself, and categorized as postnatal *qi* and the birth of *shen* (life spirit). This untainted innocence is to be protected, and as it grows and matures it still should be kept to its purest origins. This is seen in Taoist and Buddhist monks who emit a childlike persona combined with the wisdom of an elder. By nourishing you are protecting—in this case, your spirit, the eternal you, which needs guarding against physical, chemical, and emotional attack.

## Promote Vitality and Health

In simple terms, this means to make time to practice a healthy daily exercise and lifestyle regime, fully in tune with Yin and Yang and feng shui principles, meaning balanced, regular, at the same time, and in the right place.

## Longevity

Genetically, we are scheduled to live a specific period of time, as long as we follow the rules of the Tao, which sets this universal period of time. Broadly speaking, this period is somewhere between 80 and 100 years for both men and women and is classed as a long life in the context of longevity. Barring illness, accident, murder, or natural disasters, we should fulfil the programme.

## *Yangsheng* and Earth Path Connection

The Earth Path is for everyone who wishes to acquire contentment and happiness through improvements to their health and work–life balance. *Yangsheng* encompasses the specific processes you need to follow while on the path. It is the light bringer and the illuminator that allows you to see the way ahead and avoid the obstacles that would otherwise disrupt your longevity journey. Every page of this book is *yangsheng* and should provide the power source of your illumination.

# *Yangsheng* and *The Tai Chi Classics*

*The Tai Chi Classics* is the ancient textbook about how to tune in to the Tao by balancing Yin and Yang throughout the body. Within the scope of *yangsheng*, the material contained within *The Tai Chi Classics* has an important role to play, as it dwells at the heart of all things related to posture, breathing, mechanics, and *qi* circulation. (For an in-depth look at the Classics of tai chi and qigong, please refer to the author's previous book, *Healthy and Fit with Tai Chi: Perfect Your Posture, Balance, and Breathing,* published by Findhorn Press, 2015.)

The following is a brief summary of the origins of *The Tai Chi Classics*, and how to apply these Classics in the context of *yangsheng*.

## Origins and Introduction

*The Tai Chi Classics* are attributed to Chang San Feng (see Figure 31), the reputed creator of tai chi chuan, and is in simple terms an historic manual into the correct practice of tai chi. It is a head-to-toe analytical breakdown of the body (external) and how to increase the *qi* circulating through it (internal).

One of the more well-known instructions in *The Tai Chi Classics* asks the practitioner to "suspend the head as if by a string that has been attached to a cloud." This is suggested because it will raise the spirit of vitality and influence the whole body to *zhan zhang* ("stand long"), as discussed in Step 2. The string in question should theoretically be attached to the Baihui crown-point, as shown in Figure 44 in Step 7. Just this one small but significant adjustment to your resting head position will prepare you for the many beneficial mind, body, and spirit adjustments that are to come in the steps that follow.

*The Tai Chi Classics* further comments: "When the Baihui, the hundred convergence point on the crown of the head lifts, and the Yu Chen—Jade Pillow point at the base of the skull where it joints the neck stands out, then the shen (spirit of vitality) will rise to the top of the head effortlessly."

In this way, the Classics gradually work their way down the body, with the goal of creating perfection in human form, stating, "When all the Classics are in place, the body stands in natural repose."

This small introduction to the gems that are imbedded in the science of tai chi is designed to whet your appetite and give you the gift of this, the most important of all the Classics. So now you can integrate it straightaway to rejuvenate your mind and body.

Before we take the next steps, we must examine the cause and effect of premature ageing and disease, in order to avoid the pitfalls before mistakes are made, and by doing so, inform future generations.

# How to Age Prematurely

According to a census carried out by the United Nations Population Fund in 2023, the average age of life expectancy for humans is currently set at 73 years worldwide, and China and Japan, along with some Scandinavian and Mediterranean countries, still lead the way in longevity. The United Kingdom and United States do not even get a mention, despite the fact that people in the Western world are living longer due to advances in medicine (2023 figures for UK males = 81 and females = 84. USA for males = 77 and females = 82).

This worldwide average means that, in fact, many are surpassing this figure and comfortably striding into their nineties and beyond. And let us not forget the UK and USA statistics represent what you could achieve providing you live a healthy life with the full support of advanced medicine.

So, in principle, we should be expecting to live longer, and yet, how many of us know someone who has unwittingly chosen to follow a different path, one fraught with stress, frustration, limitations, and low expectations. In other words, lost.

> *Down endless paths I wander in my search for me,*
> *But each one leads to nothing, and nothing is all I see.*
>
> ~ Sifu

The words for "lost" in Chinese are *yishi de*, which can be understood to mean "lost and confused," a good description for most people taking their first tai chi and qigong classes. Yet, after only a few lessons, those who arrived lost show signs of finding themselves and exhibit an awakening of their spirit. This spiritual awakening is what the ancient Chinese call the *shen*, and in Step 7 you will learn how to open this amazing human potential.

*If you believe you can only live as long as society tells you,*
*Then your wishes will be fulfilled.*

~ Sifu

If it is generally accepted by the society you live in that women live until age 83 and men until age 81, then in your seventies, your life will be tainted and restricted by this self-fulfilling prophecy. Believing you are in the final stage of your life will change the physiology of your mind and body at a cellular level, ageing you prematurely.

The following list of causes of premature ageing may seem pretty obvious, but sometimes we need to be reminded:

- **Lack of Physical Exercise**: This leads to a body slipping into a state of stagnation.
- **Stress**: This causes self-generated inflammatory chemicals to damage the body from within.
- **Environment:** Living or lingering in toxic negative feng shui locations ages you.
- **Diet:** Poor diet is a major contributor of premature deaths. Enough said.
- **Personal Habits:** The usual culprits—smoking, drinking, drugs, and general excesses.
- **Personal Character:** Weak-spirited, domineering, obsessive, and lethargic qualities are personality flaws.
- **Poor Posture:** Many of us are oblivious to the damaging effects of poor postural alignment.

- **Poor Body Mechanics**: This refers to a body in motion that is damaging itself every time it moves.
- **Poor Breathing**: Weak respiratory function is caused by mouth breathing and poor posture.

The list could be longer, but these are the main reasons we degrade our life expectancy. They are not listed to show the most or least dangerous to you, because they all are equally hazardous to your health and wellbeing.

Men are the least likely to take regular exercise, because unlike women who gather socially and form support groups, men are often not comfortable with this type of social interaction. This can create opposing dynamics in a household, generating domestic friction and compounding problems that may already exist.

For example, a clash of personalities may occur, as we all have differing *personal character* that may impact what we like and dislike. Living in a polluted and built-up *environment* may negatively affect how we feel, as it makes us less inclined to go outdoors to exercise. When we become less physically active, the endocrine system falters, creating toxic conditions detrimental to health and affecting mood and self-esteem. Often, this can trigger negative *personal habits* in the form of comfort eating, alcohol and drug dependency, laziness, obsessiveness, and gambling. Collectively, these conditions can develop into apathy, depression, anger, and when you add *poor posture, mechanics,* and *breathing,* which most adults in modern society do not seem to understand, you have a person who is *lost.*

So what is the answer? Be more considerate towards those you love and interact with other like-minded people who are not lost and have found themselves.

## Change Elderly Perception

For many decades, it is interesting how elderly people have been perceived by society as "over the hill" or "past their best," when, in fact, we should view this stage of our lives as positively as any other stage.

Some say, "I wish I had the body of a 21-year-old but with the wisdom I have now." In some respects they are correct, so why not consider training your body to be as youthful as possible no matter what your age? To reach the age of a pensioner (currently 66 years old in the UK) and still be able to lead a fully active physical life supported by the wisdom of ages is extremely rewarding.

So it is time to change the perception of society's almost dismissive attitude to aging. In the UK, the road sign seen in Figure 8 warns the public to watch out for old people who may wander aimlessly across the highway.

**Fig. 8** UK old people road sign

But perception is everything when it comes to how society sees you and how you see yourself, because it is very true that if you think like an old person you will become old. Now let us consider what a road sign should look like if you adopt the training regime and lifestyle changes recommended in this book. The road sign should end up looking like the image depicted in Figure 9.

**Fig. 9** Revised old people road sign

# Motivation

The hurdle we must overcome to commence and sustain *yangsheng* is lack of motivation. Inspired human beings climb mountains, cross oceans, because they are driven by their mind-intent to see it through. An unexpected vision of human tenacity and admirable achievement could be all that is required to inspire and kick-start the *shen* engine in your mind. When your spirit (*shen*) is raised, you can accomplish anything.

# Ten Inspirational Research Facts about
## *Tai Chi* and *Qigong (Daoyin)*

Here is a motivational listing of medical-based health facts covering the benefits of practising *daoyin* exercises, as typically seen in Step 8. The studies tend to show more research carried out on tai chi; however, tai chi incorporates so many qigong exercises, techniques, and mechanics that it should be viewed as tai chi/qigong research.

**Tai Chi and Mind and Body**

"Tai chi improves brain metabolism and muscle energetics in older adults."[7] ~ *Journal of Neuroimaging: Official Journal of the American Society of Neuroimaging, 2018.*

Researchers confirmed that tai chi performed by an aging sample group showed significant improvements to brain metabolic and muscle recovery times after short-term tai chi training.

**Tai Chi and Cardiac Rehabilitation**

"Tai Chi is a promising exercise option for patients with coronary heart disease declining cardiac rehabilitation."[8] ~ *AHA, Journal of the American Heart Association, 2017.*

In the UK, Cardiac Kickstart, the NHS's rehabilitation unit, recommends and refers patients for tai chi and qigong classes.

## Tai Chi and Cardiovascular Disease

"Tai chi lowers blood pressure and increases the quality of life in adults with essential hypertension."[9] ~ *Heart and Lung: the American Journal of Acute and Critical Care, 2020.*

Many positive studies have been carried out in the UK and other countries throughout the world suggesting that tai chi and qigong help regulate blood pressure.

## Qigong Reduces Blood Pressure

"Qigong is an effective nonpharmacological modality to reduce blood pressure in hypertensive patients."[10] ~ *Department of Nursing, Mokpo Catholic University, South Korea, 2009.*

This is confirmation of the equal effectiveness of qigong for blood pressure issues.

## Qigong and Fibromyalgia Syndrome (FMS)

"Qigong intervention could be a useful compliment to medical treatment for subjects with FMS."[11] ~ *The Department of Clinical Psychology of Uppsala, Sweden, 2009.*

This statement was released after the clinic conducted a seven-week trial on patients with fibromyalgia (FMS).

## Tai Chi and Antibody Response

"Tai chi can increase the antibody response in older people to the flu vaccine."[12] ~ *Kinesiology Department at the University of Illinois, USA, 2007.*

Kinesiologists discovered this after a 20-week research programme. In this case, it was based on the influenza vaccine, but perhaps we can assume that it remains the same for any vaccine?

## Medical Qigong and Cancer Therapy

"Medical qigong can improve cancer patients' overall quality of life and mood status and reduce specific side effects of treatment. It may also produce physical benefits in the long term due to reduced inflammation."[13] ~ *European Society of Medical Oncologists, 2009.*

This study researched the impact of medical qigong on quality of life, fatigue, mood, and inflammation in cancer patients in a randomized controlled trial.

## Tai Chi and Heart Disease, Respiratory Disease, and Osteoarthritis

"Tai Chi is an effective exercise to help relieve potentially debilitating conditions."[14] ~ *NHS England and Public Health England, 2015.*

As a result of this acceptance by these major health authorities in the UK, tai chi and qigong are now being introduced into the mainstream clinical post-treatment therapies.

## Tai Chi and Prevention of Falls

"Tai chi may offer a superior strategy for reducing falls through its benefits of cognitive functioning."[15] ~ *The National Library of Medicine. 2020.*

In a study of 670 people with a history of falls, the group were offered tai chi sessions twice a week over six months, which lowered the fall rate by half.

## Tai Chi and Parkinson's Disease

"Tai Chi improves balance and motor control in Parkinson's disease."[16] ~ *Harvard Health (Part of Harvard University), 2013.*

Harvard Medical School in Cambridge, MA, has carried out many studies into the medical benefits of tai chi and qigong and is a leading authority in this field of study.

## Zhong-Li and Lu Discuss the Earth Path and Beyond

**Lu:** Master, why are there so few of us that seek The Way?

**Zhong-Li:** Most people do seek The Way, it's just that they aren't aware of The Way.

**Lu:** Then how can they search for something that to them doesn't exist?

**Zhong-Li:** If you were to ask them what they want in life, they would probably desire wealth, health, love, and contentment. Did we not search for the same?

**Lu:** I achieved the same when I lived amongst the masses, but realized that I yearned for more than just earthly desires, which is why I joined you here. Do I walk a different path now?

**Zhong-Li:** Fulfilling your earthly desires may make you content, but contentment alone will not satisfy the unquenchable urge in some to find the true path. You had completed the Earth Path journey, which for the majority would be enough for them to die healthy and contented. However, from the moment you chose to take the first step to my heavenly retreat here in the mountains, your path became elevated to the Middle, from where you will be able see Heaven and Earth equally.

**Lu:** So you are saying that most people will be content to walk the Earth Path and will die healthy, contented by their achievements; whereas, I and a chosen few continue our journey along new paths designed to enlighten us further.

**Zhong-Li:** Yes.

**Lu:** And what path do you tread?

**Zhong-Li:** Mine is the greatest of all paths; it is the way to The Way—never-ending but forever enlightening.

**Lu:** Then where does the Middle Path lead to?

**Zhong-Li:** Me.

# Conclusion

This first and most important tentative step along the Earth Path is accomplished by assimilating the guidance and (hopefully) inspirational facts contained in Step 1. This step can be considered as a point of awakening, a moment of realization, when our lack of vision is replaced with vision. Accordingly, it is not unusual to experience a mild sense of frustration counter-balanced by a new sense of inspiration.

*To walk into the light*
*You must first step out of the dark.*

~ Sifu

# Step 2
# *Zhang Luanli—*
# The Long Principle

The word "long" (*zhang* in Chinese) appears frequently in Chinese teaching and conversation in relation to practising and learning longevity exercises and philosophy. Over the centuries, it has grown into the next important step, which is to understand and incorporate the Long Principle in life. It stands to reason, therefore, that in the study of longevity, the concept of "long" should be understood from the ancient Chinese viewpoint. The following examples are designed to enlighten and prepare you for the next stage.

## To Live Long, You Must Stand Long

This concept is important to the creation of a body fit for longevity and is the first physical recommendation in the programme. To be correctly positioned, structurally and straight, is how to describe Stand Long posture (see Figure 10), where the feet are placed shoulder-width apart and firmly planted on the earth.

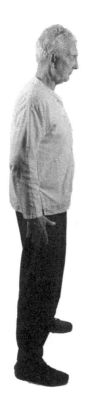

**Fig. 10** *Zhan Zhang—* Stand Long posture

At the opposite end of the body, the head must lift to connect to the sky via the crown-point (*baihui* in Chinese), with the chin gently tucked. This creates Standing Long, which is when gravity naturally aligns with the structural frame creating equilibrium and stability. To perform the posture you must endeavour to be upright, open, and relaxed, as this will release muscular tension allowing the body to naturally settle. The body is now reminiscent of the position of a car's gear stick resting in neutral. The benefits of this posture are many, as seen below, but it will take some time for your body to structurally adjust enough for you to realize and sense them. But for now, it is sufficient to have given you the task of establishing this posture.

## Benefits of Standing Long

- It equalizes the gravitational forces acting on the human frame.
- It plays a major part in retaining a good sense of balance well into later life.
- It programmes good posture as a default when the body is at rest.
- It aligns the joints of the body, reducing natural or imposed wear-and-tear.
- It allows the cardiovascular, respiratory, and mental processes to calm and centre.
- It stabilizes, bolsters, and centres the *shen* (see Step 7).

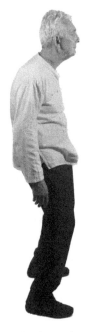

**Fig. 11** Sunken chest and rounded back posture

At the opposite end of the spectrum is the more common sunken chest, rounded back, and extended neck posture seen in Figure 11, which risks damaging the delicate discs of the spine especially in the neck. The breathing function becomes restricted as does the general circulation of the body, and if this is sustained over time it can even affect the mood. The Chinese physicians of ancient times call this an excessive Yin condition that traps the *shen* (spirit of life and vitality), creating a depressive mental state.

## To Live Long You Must Sit Long

Throughout our lives we spend a great deal of our precious time sitting, and if your seated posture is compromised for this period, a great deal of harm is caused to spine, muscular balance, organs, circulation, and breathing. The ancient (and to some extent, more recent) Chinese tended not to suffer with the back conditions seen throughout the Western world, because they would squat; whereas, the Western alternative is a soft, comfy, unsupportive chair.

For the Chinese, this would naturally rest and stretch the spinal column, when in comparison, the comfy chair option would likely cause the spine to be deformed and in compression. Even when sitting on a conventional chair, the Chinese would sit with exactly the same principles as the Stand Long structure, applied to sitting. In Figure 12, the key is to sit erect on the sitting bones (ischial tuberosities) that only protrude when squatting to sit. (Note: Sitting Long relates only to posture and not to time spent sitting; however, it is still worthwhile mentioning that you should avoid sitting for too long a period, as this will create damaging stagnation, especially in the lower body.)

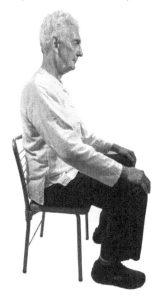

**Fig. 12** Sitting Long posture

## Benefits of Sitting Long

- It reduces the load on the spinal discs.
- It allows the pelvis to rock back and forth in harmony with the breathing.
- It keeps the brain alert, increasing concentration time.
- It helps the digestive system work.
- It helps maintain circulation between torso and legs.

The correct sitting position is shown above, but unfortunately the most commonly practised sitting method is shown in Figure 13: arms and legs crossed and body slumped, sitting on the coccyx instead of the sitting bones. Our human adoption of this unnatural sitting method compresses the spine and its discs and restricts circulation in the legs. The breathing function is also suppressed, due to the thoracic spine being bowed and fixed; the ribcage is likewise held and fixed by the arms and slumped posture.

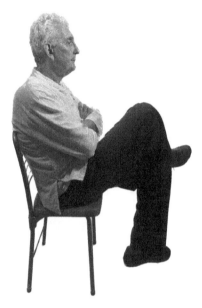

**Fig. 13** Slumped sitting

Note: A good posture maxim to remember at this juncture is, "Sit as you would stand, and stand as you would sit." When sitting long there is less impact on the spinal discs, and leg circulation is not compromised due to the sitting bones elevating the soft tissues of the pelvis and thighs, allowing good blood flow. You will also notice how much easier it is to breathe, and by sitting alert, you will remain alert.

## To Live Long, You Must Breathe Long

Sound advice on correct breathing echoes from China's ancient past and involves what is known as "breathing long." What is long breathing? What are its benefits? And how do you do it safely and sensibly?

## Benefits of Long Breathing

- It releases hidden, suppressed, and pent-up emotions within seconds.
- It switches on the parasympathetic nervous system, allowing you to rest and digest.
- It regulates the heart, high blood pressure, and asthma.
- It trains the diaphragm to operate at its optimum level, which helps the circulation of blood through the core of the body, and as such is considered a second heart.

For more on "breathing long," refer to Steps 3 and 8, which cover in more detail practical training in long breathing through specific exercises and High Chest Shallow Mouth Breathing (HCSMB), a common breathing dysfunction.

> *To experience* fangsung *in mind and*
> *body, let the breath lead the way.*
> ~ Sifu

## To Live Long, You Must Walk Long

There was a singer from Ireland called Val Doonican, who, in 1965, released a record called "Walk Tall." Its lyrics contained wise words, "Walk tall, walk straight, and look the world right in the eye." He goes on to say, "That's what my mama told me when I was about knee high." The lyrics of the song carry a Celtic flavouring that likely came from their deep and rich cultural history, and their message resonates equally with that of the ancient Chinese.

Tall (long) in this instance relates to maintaining an upright, fully extended posture, eyes firmly fixed on the horizon and a positive walking action that comes from, and is coordinated by, all four limbs remaining relaxed and naturally extended. "Walking long" also means walking for a long period and distance; however, time and distance covered is relative and should be dictated by your physical ability.

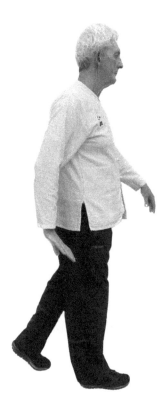

**Fig. 14** Long Walking Posture

If you are inspired to start a walking programme, you should make sure you have the correct walking shoes and clothing. Your first steps should last no more than 10 minutes (five minutes there and five minutes back) at a medium strolling pace on a flat surface, then gradually increase this over a few weeks to a 30-minute programme (15 minutes there and 15 minutes back). When you are confident your stamina and general health has improved, you should gradually introduce routes with inclines and vary the surface type from flat (smooth) to hilly (undulating). This will improve your sense of balance (proprioception) and deliver many health benefits. Figure 14 shows a relaxed, fully extended walking posture that, if adopted, can be life-enhancing for your physical and mental health.

# Walking Quietly *(Zuochan Xingchan)*

In the development of perfect walking, it is important to always "walk with the Tao," which is different from gravitationally aligned long walking. This is called "walking quietly" (*zuochan xingchan*) and is when your steps become so light you are unnoticed as you approach someone.

The intensity with which the heel touches the ground as you step forward can often be so heavy it becomes audible and can detrimentally rebound forces up into the body, damaging knees, hips, and spine. It is, therefore, important to step lightly and quietly, moving with the natural grace that comes with long walking.

The three ideal frequencies for walking are: *Free and Easy Wandering* (slow, relaxed, meditative strolling for mental health, perhaps along a riverbank); *Middle Path* (normal-paced daily walking for general health), and *Extended Stride Pattern* (fast-paced walking, with short bursts for cardiovascular and respiratory health).

In contrast with the healthy long walking shown opposite, you should at all costs avoid the damaging walking posture shown in Figure 15.

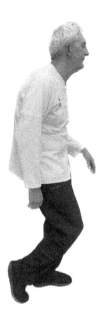

**Fig. 15** Slumped walking posture

Walking with a slumped posture not surprisingly causes the same damage as found in slumped sitting, and even damages the leg circulation, as if you have been incorrectly sitting. This is due to the knees (circulation and mechanical enhancers) remaining slightly bent throughout the action.

The unnatural posture and motion discourages the natural heel-to-toe rolling action of the feet and replaces it with a flat-footed, almost shuffling action. If you lose the springy tendon heel-to-toe rolling action of the feet, joints stiffen, circulation stagnates, and foot-pounding percussion radiates upwards throughout the body, increasing potential damage to all of the joints involved in motion, including the spine (other than that, it is perfectly fine).

## Benefits of Long Walking

- It maintains your youthful, springy tendons, which operate as shock absorbers and walking accelerators.
- It regulates circulation throughout the body.
- It regulates cardiovascular and respiratory functions.
- It lifts the mood by releasing positive endorphins.
- It maintains a good sense of balance.

According to the American Heart Association, walking has the following health benefits:[17]

- It has the lowest dropout of any physical activity.
- Thirty minutes a day reduces the risk of coronary disease.
- It improves blood pressure.
- It regulates blood sugar levels.
- It reduces the risk of osteoporosis and breast and colon cancer.
- You will gain two hours of life for each hour walked.

There are three other long principles that also form important facets of human life: long thinking, long moving, and long eating.

## To Live Long, You Must Think Long

"Thinking long" does not mean thinking for a long time, as over-thinking damages the spleen; instead, it relates to how you perceive your life expectancy. If you are told by public mortality statistics that men have a life expectancy of say 80 years and women 83 years, and you believe this to be true, you can expect your body at a cellular level to degenerate the closer you get to the end-game figure. The message, therefore, is to "think long" beyond society's expectations. Visualize and believe that 100 years is comfortably achievable, and this will slow the rate of degeneration, keeping you younger and healthier for longer.

## To Live Long, You Must Move Long

Moving long is called "Healthy Living Form," which means you must incorporate natural body mechanics in all your everyday mundane movements. You should bend, extend, coil, recoil, fold, unfold, and twist to avoid stiffness in the joints and soft tissues, with the ultimate aim of dodging life-threatening stagnation.

The key is to never lose the natural postures and elasticity that we enjoyed in our youth. If you do that, you will have achieved Healthy Living Form.

## To Live Long, You Must Eat Long

This is probably the most obvious of all the "long" maxims. Quite simply, to "eat long" means to take your time when eating. To do that, you must chew "long," meaning that small amounts of food placed in the mouth should be chewed slowly and, depending on the choice of food, savoured. This allows more time for the essential enzymes in saliva to break down the solids, making it easier to digest and helping maintain a healthy digestive system.

## Zhong-Li and Lu Discuss "Long"

**Lu:** Master, you often mention and include "long" in our conversations. Why is this?

**Zhong-Li:** How can any conversation not at some time include "long"? "Long" is embedded in the fabric of our lives, and if considered in the context of challenges to the human spirit of discovery and adventure, "long" is greeted with great respect and seen as a milestone of achievement.

**Lu:** I see. So, when you say the three paths to the Tao are "long," do we need to view the completion of each path as a milestone?

**Zhong-Li:** Without these achievement markers, it can feel like the journey or personal challenge may never end. However, as you reach each milestone along the way, in your mind you are reassured that *more* is in fact becoming *less*.

**Lu:** So, "long" does not necessarily mean the desired goal will take a long time to materialize?

**Zhong-Li:** If you apply yourself to the Long Principle in body, mind, and spirit, your perceived "long" journey turns out to be but a mere step.

**Lu:** Now I understand. So those who seek the Tao without embracing "long" may never complete the journey.

**Zhong-Li:** Yes.

## Conclusion

The human body is constructed so that to function properly it must be kept upright, open, and relaxed. Hopefully, the information in Step 2 has clarified how to achieve this, and you are clear in your mind about why following the Long Principle is essential to longevity. It is an important stepping stone along the way to a long and fulfilled life.

# Step 3
## *Shen Huxi—*
## Profound Breathing

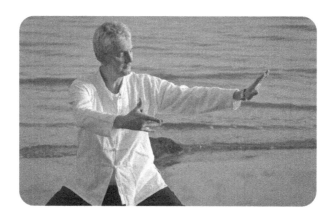

Breathing is the most important human function you will experience in your lifetime. It is the first thing you do when you are born and the last thing you do when you die. How you embrace this life-giving and supporting gift in between birth and death will determine whether you enjoy a healthy, fulfilled life or a disappointing uphill struggle.

Step 3 will discuss the causes and symptoms of High Chest Shallow Mouth Breathing (HCSMB), supported by some medical facts highlighting the damage this type of dysfunctional breathing causes. In addition, you will learn how to gradually transform your breathing mechanics from insufficient to profound, by following the guidance of the ancient Chinese Taoist physicians.

# What is *Shen Huxi?*

The Chinese word *shen* when coupled with *huxi* means "profound breathing," but on its own, in the Taoist arts, it can mean, "mysteriously deep" and "spirit," correlated to strength of mind, willpower, and character.

In Step 7, we will explore *shen* in a broader context, but in Step 3, you will get your first taste of its "deep and spiritual" meaning. On its own, the word *huxi* is used to relate to your breathing generally, not specifically. Placing the word *huxi* after *shen* lifts it to new and interesting levels. As noted by Grandmaster Dr. Yang, Jwing-Ming: *Shen huxi* means "spirit" and "breathing in harmony."[18]

Here in the West, with the exception of the medical fraternity, we see breathing as just something we do that is part of living. In the Far East, by contrast, breathing is seen as deep and meaningful, the most important thing we humans do, and is referred to as "profound." In the Chinese mind, *huxi is* profound due to the way it affects health, both positively and negatively, depending on how you embrace it. In addition, ancient Chinese warriors and healers used the power of the breath (*jing qi*) to enhance their warrior prowess and healing effectiveness, respectively.

In Chinese, the word *qi* can mean "air" or "rice" and is considered quintessential to life—we breathe the air and eat the rice in order to live. Here, we will stay focused on air, as it is the primary life support and source of your body's vital energy. By breathing correctly and meaningfully, health blossoms, and if this vital function is compromised in some way, the first thing to suffer is your health and vitality. Insufficient breathing manifests internally as a lack of vitality and motivation, and visually as a pale sickly complexion. In the minds of the ancients, *shen huxi* meant "breathing that reinforces health, vitality, mental strength *(shen)*, and wards off your enemies (disease)," so you can understand why it was considered "profound."

# Cause and Effect of HCSMB

Some people develop a type of dysfunctional shallow breathing known as High Chest Shallow Mouth Breathing (HCSMB) that can seriously damage health. If you try to "breathe long" with HCSMB, you will find it almost impossible, because as long as the structural imbalances in your body core remain, just attempting to "breathe long" will feel as though an unseen hand is gripping your diaphragm. Not a pleasant sensation.

To relieve HCSMB, you must first release internal stresses (physical and mental) that caused the restricted breathing in the first place by introducing the eight *daoyin* (physical restorations) balanced with *jing zuo* (mental restorations) into your life. Together, they will positively alter the negative dynamics.

Newborn babies instinctively breathe "long" and profoundly, which means they are naturally nose-breathers. This is supported by deep, long, abdominal respiration, which encourages their diaphragm to fully sink into the lower abdominal cavity on inhalation and spring back up fully into the chest cavity on exhalation. This is the desired way.

Unfortunately, as they get older (usually from about the age of eight onwards), some youngsters drift away from the Tao, and so begins a life potentially limited by self-inflicted health problems.

Sadly, in our age of social media, children are spending too much time bent over their computer screens or smartphones, and this is where the seeds of HCSMB are sown. By fixing their thoracic spine in a bent position (see the slumped, bowed-outward spine depicted in Figure 15), they are switching off not one but all three of the Three Essential Mechanics of natural healthy breathing: thoracic spine, ribcage, and pelvis. These must move as one for the body to enjoy full and healthy respiration. Furthermore, when one of the three is held fixed and not allowed to move, the other two freeze simultaneously.

*Respiration involves the absorption of oxygen and the emission of carbon dioxide, both to and from the lungs.*

- Sifu

The net result is to restrict the chest cavity expansion and contraction, and the diaphragm from sinking then springing fully back up. At this stage, natural nose breathing is unable to feed enough essential oxygen to the cells of the body and, most importantly, the brain. Consequently, the brain senses this shortage and directs the mouth to open to make up for the shortfall, even though this never works while the posture is out of structural alignment.

This hollow-chested posture tends to concentrate the breathing to the back of the lungs, leaving the side and front underutilized. By releasing the thoracic spine, the whole surface area of the lungs can be engaged, helping conditions associated with Chronic Obstructive Pulmonary Disease (COPD).

There are many other reasons your breathing can be adversely affected by HCSBM; for example, nasal airway obstructions caused by allergies, nasal polyps, sinusitis, and physical deformity. The other obvious self-inflicted cause of HCSBM is smoking, which clogs up the alveoli air sacs in the lungs, where vital respiration takes place, leading to low oxygen intake and low carbon release. In exactly the same way as described above for fixed posture condition, the brain calls for more oxygen by opening the mouth.

# The Three Essential Mechanics of Breathing

## 1. Thoracic Spine Flexion and Extension

This is called bowing inwards (extension) and bowing outwards (flexion) and correlates exactly to the breathing: bowing inwards = breathing inwards, and bowing outwards = breathing outwards. To ensure you are creating the conditions for your thoracic spine to engage with your breathing, you must ensure that your head is always maintained in an upward-lifting position from the crown-point, as seen in figures 10, 12, and 14. This centres the spine generally and delivers all of its three sections (cervical, thoracic, and lumbar) into the mechanism of breathing.

## 2. Ribcage Expansion and Contraction

The bowing action of the thoracic spine directly impacts the thorax (chest) by flaring the ribcage open when bowing inward and folding it to close when bowing outward. This directly assists the lungs to position correctly in the chest cavity to operate its healthy gas exchange and helps drive the diaphragm.

## 3. Pelvic Tilting

In the three positions of the pelvis seen in Figure 16, all three work in unison to prompt and maximize the full and necessary range of movement (ROM) of the thoracic spine and ribcage action. Pelvic tilting mechanically opens the abdomen (inhalation) to create space for the diaphragm to lower, and also closes and contracts the abdomen (exhalation), directing the diaphragm to rise and return into the chest cavity.

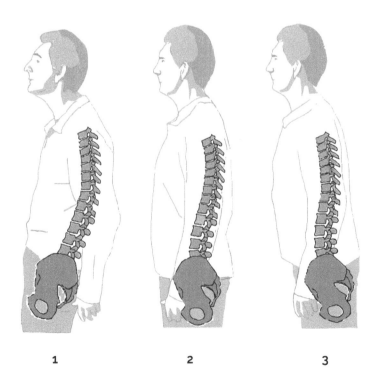

1                    2                    3

**Fig. 16** Pelvic tilting and breathing

*Number 1 (Thoracic Spine Flexion)* equates to an outward breath with thoracic spine naturally bowing outward and ribcage folding inward (exhalation).

*Number 2 (Ribcage Expansion and Contraction)* is the neutral midway pivotal point between breathing in or out, and where the spine and torso are at rest and gravitationally aligned. Note: This position should never remain fixed and, in fact, the desired condition for healthy breathing is when all three are kept in perpetual motion (even when sleeping).

*Number 3 (Pelvic Tilting)* opens the ribs, thorax, and airways and bows the thoracic spine inwards (inhalation).

> *In order to balance energy,*
> *you must first balance the breath.*
>
> ~ Tai chi maxim

Remember: Two-thirds of your breathing comes from your diaphragm, and the other third comes from your chest cavity (thoracic spine and ribcage, combined).

## Reasons Why HCSBM Is Not Recommended

- It weakens the efficient function of the deep respiratory muscles, especially the diaphragm.
- It introduces shallow breathing mechanics, weakening the whole respiratory function (gas exchange).
- It dries up the Sweet Dew (saliva), causing increased bacteria growth.
- It creates a respiration imbalance that can release too much $CO_2$, causing hyperventilation.
- It increases the risk of asthma attack by constricting the smooth muscles around the airways.

- It allows contaminated air directly into the lungs, bypassing the filtering process of the nose.
- It can increase the risk of developing chronic nasal conditions, because the nose eventually switches its air filtration and decontamination systems off due to underusage.
- It increases the chance of developing COPD, when the nose becomes redundant and the breathing only relies on the mouth.

# Remedial Actions

Here is a list of important practical actions designed to reintroduce longevity breathing and eliminate HCSMB.

- First follow all the posture advice given in this step.
- Wear loose-fitting clothing, especially around the waist.
- Gradually retrain your breathing from mouth to the nose.
- Practise sitting quietly (*jing zuo*), with good posture and breathing through the nose.
- Avoid breathwork if you are overtired, under the influence of drugs and alcohol, emotionally charged, or have eaten a heavy meal.
- Breathe in and out in harmony with the mechanics of the Three Essentials.
- Be aware of the chin swinging up (out) and down (in) as you breathe in and out, respectively.
- Maintain open armpits, as this helps the Three Essentials to function.
- Start with eight breathing cycles, and increase gradually to 24 over a few weeks.
- When the abdomen feels like it is expanding and contracting like a balloon inflating and deflating, your foundation and recovery is in place.
- Breathing in should become natural and effortless. Breathing out should feel like you are just letting go.

# The White Crane and Its Influence on Exercise and Breathing

When tai chi and qigong masters talk of longevity and breathing, they more often than not refer to the majestic White Cranes of Longevity or the Prince of All Birds, as they are known. In classic Taoist tradition, the ancient Chinese were adept at observing nature in all its majesty, and among the myriad of creatures, the red-crowned white crane stood out as inspirational and exceptional.

Historically, the Chinese respected any creatures displaying grace, beauty, and spirit, all of which are embodied in the red-crowned white crane. Standing five feet tall and adopted as a native species in China, despite also residing in Japan and Korea, this crane has become known as the Manchurian crane. They symbolically represent:

- **Longevity:** They have been known to live as long as 100 years, were linked to long life through their roles as conveyances of the immortals, and their white feathers were likened to the colour of elderly people's hair.
- **Loyalty:** They mate for life.
- **Strength:** They can fly great distances (some are known to fly 2,000 miles).
- **Mythology:** In Taoist arts, they are believed to be intermediaries of the Heavenly Immortals, because they carry the souls of the dead to the heavens.
- **Nobility:** Their symbols were (and still are) adorned on the clothing of *fang shih* (Taoist priests) and other members of Chinese high office (see Figure 17).
- **Purity:** Their pristine white feathers reflect purity and innocence.
- **Grace:** Their general movements, coupled with their mating and bonding dance, carry an elegance and balletic beauty that has been assimilated into tai chi and qigong.

- **Spirit:** They ferociously defend their territory and chicks (colts) from predators and are themselves top-level predators.
- **Balance:** They can sustain their balance while standing on a single bamboo shoot during high winds.
- **Rarity:** Red-crowned white cranes are the second rarest of the crane species; only the whooping crane surpasses them.
- **Luck:** By adorning your house, clothing, or place of work with their symbolism, they represent good luck and prosperity.
- **Wisdom:** Cranes are very intelligent birds and, as such, represent wisdom and knowledge.
- **Harmony:** They are the embodiment of Yin and Yang harmony due to their interaction with one another and how they mate for life.

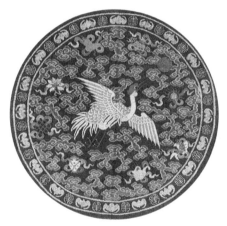

**Fig. 17** Qing dynasty badge of office

The elegant, flowing and graceful expressions of the red-crowned white crane were observed by inquisitive Taoist recluses, who discovered that by mimicking its movements they felt heathier and more energized. In Step 8, the elegance, spirit, and mechanics of these movements permeate most of the longevity exercises and can be experienced personally. Consequently, over many centuries a system of self-defence and therapeutic exercise (*daoyin*/qigong) has evolved in China known as White Crane Kung Fu. This martial art solely concentrates on the nature of the red-crowned white crane, which has gained respect worldwide.

# White Crane Shapes Have Meaning

The crane seen in Figure 18 is typical of the subtle messages encrypted into paintings of that era: The crane is gazing at the heavens pondering its magnitude and secrets. In terms of exercise and breathing, the shapes that cranes make are profound, deep, and meaningful, which is why it is important at this step to highlight two key shapes for healthy breathing:

## 1. White Crane Airs Its Wings

In Figure 19, the majestic crane spreads its wings in such a fashion as to energize them and fill its lungs to prepare for flight, while lifting its head and expanding its chest.

In Figure 20, this tai chi posture is called White Crane Airs Its Wings, and is to be performed in the same way as the actual crane—by lifting the top of the head and opening the chest while spreading the arms apart. This is the shape for inhalation.

This is by far the most famous of all tai chi postures and should be performed in the spirit of the crane:

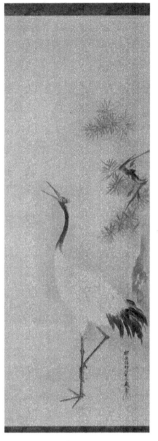

**Fig. 18**

Heaven-gazing crane

- Whether it is a single foot or both feet planted firmly on the earth, you should feel the whole body stabilized by the immense force of earth *qi* residing underfoot.
- Any replication of the crane's wing action must first emanate up from the feet and express itself through to the wing tips.
- The connection between the legs and the wings is the spine, which must interpret the rising power from the legs and direct it into the arms (wings).

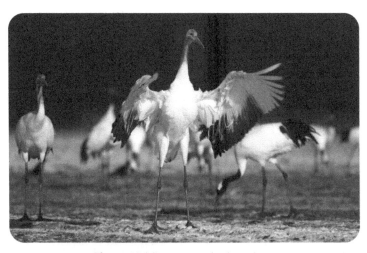

**Fig. 19** White crane airs its wings

In Step 8, you will find a detailed description of how to perform this powerful, therapeutic breathing routine (see *Bai He Shenkai*—White Crane Stretching).

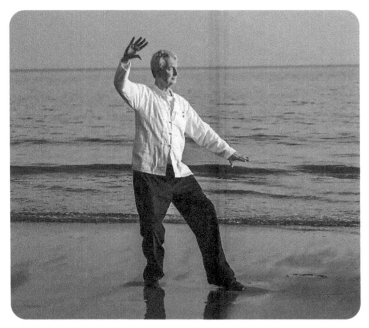

**Fig. 20** Tai chi version of White Crane Airs Its Wings

## 2. The Landing Crane

In Figure 21, the wing shapes are partially closing and lowering as the cranes approach the earth in just the same way as we see aeroplanes coming in to land.

In Figure 22, this qigong posture is also called Landing Crane and is for grounding and earthing mind and body. This is the shape for exhalation.

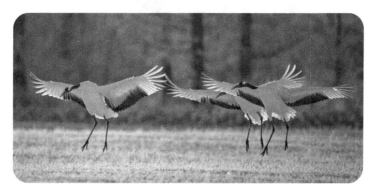

**Fig. 21** Landing cranes

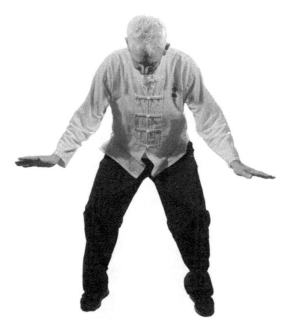

**Fig. 22** Qigong version of Landing Crane

**Notes**

When they are combined harmoniously, the movements of White Crane Airs Its Wings and Landing Crane form the classic breathing trainer and respiratory therapy called Flying Crane. Benefits attributed to White Crane breathing (Profound Long Breathing) are that it extends the lungs/diaphragm downwards, and by doing so massages the organs, aiding digestion and easing constipation.

# Three-Stage Breathing

### 1. Turtle Neck Breathing *(Wugui-bozi Huxi)*

You should lift the head up just as the turtle does in extending its neck in an upward arc. This shape opens the airways, blood vessels, nerve pathways, and cervical spine—all combining to maximize the flow of oxygen to the brain. Inhale through the nose when performing.

Following this you should lift the crown of the head as you tuck your chin gently. This creates the perfect conditions for your airways to expel carbon dioxide from your lungs. In addition, this head position correctly aligns the cervical neck joints and supporting soft tissues. You must exhale through the nose.

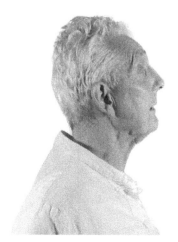 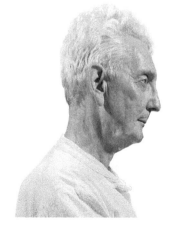

**Fig. 23** Turtle Neck (inhale)     **Fig. 24** Turtle Neck (exhale)

## 2. Crane Breathing *(Bai He Huxi)*

Crane Breathing involves the bowing in and out of the thoracic spine primarily, but in fact integrates the whole spine and body. Cranes charge their lungs (inhaling) by inward bowing of their spines and outward bowing when exhaling. This natural process increases their lung capacity by expanding their chest cavity, and it works exactly the same for humans.

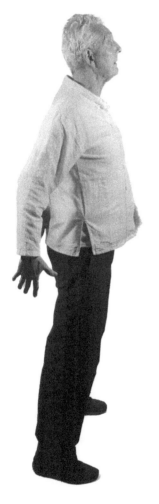 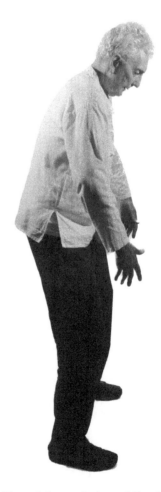

**Fig. 25** Crane Inward Bowing (inhale)   **Fig. 26** Crane Outward Bowing (exhale)

**Notes**

- Turtle Neck breathing must be incorporated into the spine-bowing action to make sure all the mechanics of breathing are unified in a single action.
- If you have any spine conditions that limit its range of motion, you must reduce the movement to a safer, more comfortable range.
- To practise these routines, you should perform no more than eight repetitions at any one time.

## 3. Dragon Breathing *(Long Huxi)*

When you combine Turtle Neck with Crane breathing and add long spine-wave, you have Dragon breathing. In fact, the mechanics of this profound method involve the whole body, from toes to fingertips. When operating effortlessly and naturally, you will have developed the ultimate level of breathing: *ti huxi* (whole-body breathing).

The dragon symbolically represents:

- The Lord of the Heavens
- The keeper of the Tao and The Way itself
- The bringer of rain
- The Chinese emperor
- Waves and clouds
- Males
- Sagehood
- Wisdom

People born in the Year of the Dragon are thought to be bestowed with grace, power, wealth, good fortune, and longevity. Dragons represent superior human beings who exhibit the virtues and characteristics of Heaven. The Dragon's home is thought to be in lakes and oceans.

**Note:** The details of *ti huxi* will be covered in a later book.

# Five Key Characteristics of *Shen Huxi*

## 1. Calm *(Jing)*

Listen to your breathing. If it is hardly audible, then you have calm breathing, created by a calm mind and a relaxed body, free from muscular tension that would otherwise tense the breathing.

## 2. Slender *(Xi)*

By maintaining and developing nose breathing until it has returned to being natural and effortless, you will experience "slender breathing": The inhalation and exhalation flows finely and not like a torrent.

## 3. Deep *(Shen)*

The deep centre line of the body lies just in front of the inside face of the spine. This is your gravitational core, where the breathing should be sensed in order to centre itself. In this location, the breathing naturally expands the chest cavity equally in all directions, allowing the lungs to be placed centrally in the thoracic cavity and the diaphragm to operate through its centre, creating a full range of motion and a powerful respiration.

## 4. Long *(Zhang)*

Your sense of breathing inward should reach down to your lower abdomen (and even be sensed touching the pelvic floor), which is the home of your life-force *qi.* If the breathing occurs in this location naturally, you have developed Embryonic Breathing; that is, returned to the most natural state of "long breathing." In the same way as deep breathing, the breath should be sensed expanding in all directions as if inflating a ball.

## 5. Continuous *(You)*

This key component comes last after you have accomplished the first four characteristics listed above. Only when calm, slender, deep, and long are operating in perfect harmony will continuous breathing becomes established. This deeply refined state of breathing ensures your respiration is consistently working at its optimum efficiency, servicing the cells throughout the whole body (*ti huxi*).

# Ten Inspirational Facts about Profound Breathing

- Exhaling through the nose controls the volume of air released in such a way that oxygen remains longer in the lungs for increased extraction, resulting in the availability of 10–20 percent more oxygen.
- Nose breathing creates correct oxygen–carbon dioxide exchange, so the blood will maintain a balanced PH.
- Non-profound mouth breathing causes the brain to think carbon dioxide is being lost too quickly, so it inadvertently makes the airways produce more mucus, blocking the nasal passages, and causing the chest to wheeze. This unnaturally slows down the breathing and makes it shallow and constricts the blood vessels, thereby raising blood pressure.
- Consciously nose breathing during the day is more likely to lead to it continuing subconsciously overnight.
- Scientists have noted that the capacity and function of the lungs doubles when practising nose (profound) breathing.
- The combination of correct posture and nose breathing drives the diaphragm downward. This compresses the adrenal glands, which release health-enhancing metabolic hormones.
- The natural funnelling effect of nose breathing helps maintain lung elasticity.
- In Chinese Traditional Medicine, it is said that when the lung *qi* (diaphragm) descends (profound breathing), the function of the large intestine is normal and bowel movement free.
- In connection with fact number 8 above, the ancients said, "The atmosphere (gases) of the lungs cannot be harvested (exchanged) when the lower burner space (lower abdominal cavity) is blocked."
- Profound breathing is The Way of the newborn child, and although humans physically change as they grow into adulthood and beyond, The Way of the child should remain.

## Zhong-Li and Lu Discuss Profound Breathing

**Lu:** Master, we have just walked up a very steep incline to get to this resting place, and my breathing is laboured when yours is calm and unaffected. Why is this?

**Zhong-Li:** This is because your breathing still carries the weight of your previous life among the masses.

**Lu:** But I am fit and strong, and yet in comparison to you, I still had to breathe heavily to get here. How can I become more like you?

**Zhong-Li:** In your mind you think you have to *do* something to be like me, when in fact you would be wiser to do *nothing* to be like me.

**Lu:** Are you saying I can't *make* my breathing longer and calmer?

**Zhong-Li:** Your breathing is a gift from the Tao, and it is said that those who seek the Tao will never find the Tao. But if you merge with the Tao by *non-doing*, the Tao will be found.

**Lu:** Are you saying my profound breathing is already here within me and by doing nothing I unleash it?

**Zhong-Li:** Yes.

# Conclusion

Steps 1, 2, and 3 lay a foundation for your understanding of how to make the necessary changes to your mind, posture, mechanics, and most importantly, breathing. The next steps are where you broaden your knowledge of how to achieve health and longevity. To do this, you must ensure that you are motivated. Step 4 is designed to provide inspiration and wisdom from longevity icons of the past, and you could say this is where legend meets fact.

# Step 4
# Secrets of the Longevity Icons

This chapter tells the stories of several legendary figures and deities from ancient times and the recent past who lived up to the doctrines of the Tao and succeeded in living long and dying healthy. These long-lived mortals, both real and fictional, observed a regime that allowed them to lengthen their lifespan.

Through their practices, they evolved from adepts to Lohans to real people to rainbow beings to immortals and finally, celestial gods. They leave a valuable legacy, and their individual journeys have something to say to us today from which we can perhaps gain inspiration.

This section also examines Chinese symbolism as a way of helping you understand the veneration of longevity in culturally rich China.

## Shou Lao

The Taoist figure Shou Lao stands out as one of the premier deities of Chinese culture. As the Chinese god of longevity, his blessing is believed to bestow a long and healthy life. He is said to have lived some time during the Han Dynasty (206 BC–AD 220), and legend states that he was born old and went on to become a god that personifies Canopus, the second brightest star in the Southern Hemisphere, also known as Sirius. Due to this association, he is also called Nan Gi Lou Ren (old Man of the South Pole).

He is also often seen as one of the Three Celestial Stars: *Shou Lao* (Longevity), *Luxing* (Prosperity), and *Fuxing* (Happiness). Shou Lao, Zhong-Li, and Ancestor Lu are part of a group known as the Eight Immortals, forming the most famous deities in Chinese folklore history.

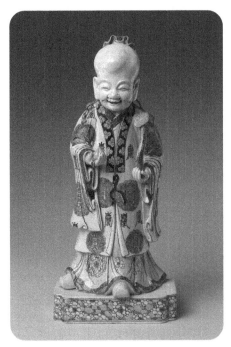

**Fig. 27** Shou Lao, with peach

In Figure 27, Shou Lao is holding a peach in his right hand and a gourd in his left. The peach is known as the fruit of immortality while the gourd carries the elixir of immortality.

The symbols associated with Shou Lou can be summarized as follows:

- **Large Head, Long Earlobes, and Long, White Beard**: These attributes represent a person of great age and accumulated wisdom (*chih*).
- **Deer:** Deer are believed to be able to find an immortality-granting fungus.
- **Cranes:** Cranes convey the immortals on their backs (see Step 3).
- **Staff:** Shou Lao's staff is made of peach wood and depicts reverence in old age.
- **Bats**: Symbolically, five bats (*wu fu*) represent the five blessings of longevity and dying healthy: long life, good health, wealth, virtue, and a peaceful death.
- **Pine Trees:** Pine trees were especially revered by the ancient Chinese. During the Qin Dynasty (221–206 BC), the 1st Emperor bestowed the rank of "Mandarin of the 5th Class" on an ancient pine tree on the sacred mountain of Tai Shan, because this tree had repeatedly survived the harshest winters and never lost its needles. Since then, the pine tree has been associated with longevity.
- **Peaches:** In Traditional Chinese Medicine (TCM), peaches are used to treat circulatory heart conditions and many other ailments that affect the elderly. Since early Chinese history, peaches have been thought to contain life-extending properties and have been associated with health and longevity.
- **Dragon:** In many Shou Lao images, you will see a carved dragon's head atop his peach-wood staff. As noted earlier, the dragon is known as the Lord of the Heavens, and people born in the Year of the Dragon are thought to be bestowed with grace, power, wealth, good fortune, and longevity.
- **Children:** Children symbolize Youthful Spirit of Vitality and Innocence required in the pursuit of longevity. Shou Lao is also often depicted with a young child confirming the maxim from the Taoist art of Tai Chi Chuan: "Through the practice of tai chi, you will develop the strength of a lumberjack and the spirit, vitality, and suppleness of a child."

# The First Yellow Emperor, Huang Di

Huang Di ruled from 2697 to 2597 BC and was believed to have lived to 111 years due to his Taoist lifestyle. He is said to have devised a sequence of exercises for the general population to practise daily, comprising yogic postures, flowing silk-like movements, "long diaphragm"–generated breathing techniques, and inner gazing to raise self and spiritual awareness. Taken together, these disciplines constituted the first signs of *daoyin* (qigong) exercises taking shape in early China.

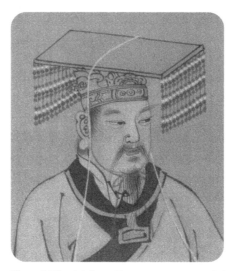

**Fig. 28** The Yellow Emperor—Huang Di

The Chinese classic *Nei Ching*, written around the third century BC and commonly known as *The Yellow Emperor's Classic of Internal Medicine*, is based on a dialogue between Emperor Huang Di and Ch'i Po, divine Tao teacher and advisor to his court. In one exchange, the two discuss longevity:

> **Huang Di:** "I have heard that people of antiquity lived for over 100 years, and yet they remained active and did not become decrepit in their activities." He then questioned: "Why are people nowadays becoming decrepit and failing, reaching only half that age?"

**Ch'i Po replied:** "In ancient times people understood how to live in accord with the Tao (the source and root of everything that makes up the known universe), and they patterned themselves upon Yin and Yang (the two destructive and creative forces of the Tao)."[19]

In order to live long like the ancients that Ch'i Po referred to, he recommended the following:[20]

- **Adjust your life to accord with Yin and Yang.** (See Step 5)
- **Escape the cold, and seek the warmth.** Avoid too much exposure to extreme temperatures, especially in the winter.
- **Moderate eating and drinking.** Over-indulgence will shorten your life and raise the potential for dying sickly.
- **The hours of rising and retiring are to be regular.** Listen to your body clock (see Step 5).
- **Avoid weaknesses and noxious influences.** Drugs, alcohol, gambling, and toxic people.
- **Avoid injurious winds.** Winds that come from a specific direction, especially in winter, that carry winter-borne illnesses.
- **Exercise restraint of the will.** Uncontrolled emotions damage the spirit (*shen*), such as excessive sadness or excessive anger (see Step 7).
- **Overcome excessive desires.** Craving, greed, lust, and obsessiveness will damage the wisdom mind (*chih yi*) and leave you open to irrational, unguided decisions.
- **Do not overwork.** With a mind and body in tune with the Tao, you should be able to toil and not get too weary. Follow the three rhythms of daily life: work, rest, and play, and enjoy a *yangsheng* life.

Ch'i Po then makes the following bold and important statement on longevity:

> *These men [who abide by the above advice] can be called pure of heart. They could live for more than one hundred years and remain active without becoming decrepit, because their virtue was perfect and never imperilled.*[21]

# Lao Tzu

Another Taoist icon is Lao Tzu (Old Master), who in Taoist circles is regarded as the founding father of Taoism. Yet another iconic figure in the same mould as King Arthur, he is more mythical than factual and yet, like Arthur, he lives on in the minds of his people with god-like status.

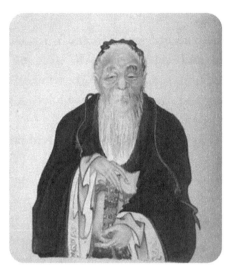

**Fig. 29** Lao Tzu

According to D.C. Lau, translator of the 1963 edition of the *Tao Te Ching*, Lao Tzu's works consist of sayings that embody a kind of wisdom associated with old age (longevity). Lao Tzu is reputed to have lived sometime around the 6th century BC and worked as an archivist in the court of the Zhou Dynasty (1046–256 BC). Having become disgruntled with the way society and its rulers behaved, in true Taoist tradition he escaped to the sacred mountains in search of enlightenment.

The next time he surfaces, riding on a water buffalo/ox and aged 150–200 years old, is to bestow his academic masterpiece, the *Tao Te Ching (The Book of The Way and Its Virtue)*. During the middle of the 2nd century BC, after China had become unified under Emperor Qin Shi Huang, founder of the Qin Dynasty (221–206 BC), the *Tao Te Ching* became an established sourcebook of wisdom at the imperial court.

More so than any other historic Chinese sage, Lao Tzu's literary legacy endures to this day and influences people from all walks of life.

The sample of the *Tao Te Ching* manuscript shown in Figure 30 was unearthed by archaeologists in a tomb in Mawangdui, Hunan Province, and is described as being ink on silk. It is from this Taoist classic that the following guidance is abstracted to help guide us on our longevity mission:[22]

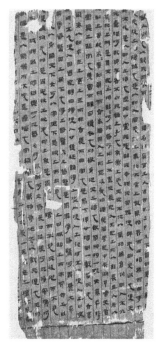

**Fig. 30**

*Tao Te Ching* manuscript

- **Live without possessiveness, act without presumption.** In times gone by, when people had few possessions, it was easy to live without possessiveness. They accepted their place in life and just got on with it. Now, however, in this greedy materialistic world, this doctrine is needed more than ever.
- **In life be wary, as one crossing a swollen river in the winter.** The ancient warriors lived with an awareness of their enemies. They were always conscious of their surroundings, as if they expected to be ambushed by assailants. By doing so, they retained sharp, clear minds and bodies, thereby avoiding the dulling of the senses that comes with complacency.
- **Relax like ice at the melting point.** This is another way of describing the requisite state of mind needed to achieve *yangsheng* and navigate the Earth Path. This aura of calmness and tranquillity is called *fangsung*, which literally translates to "relax and let go." The combination of tai chi/qigong exercise and *jing zuo* meditation naturally introduces this deep sense of stillness within.
- **Be as simple as an uncarved wooden block.** No airs, no graces, no ego—just simplicity, humbly journeying through life below the

radar, in tune with the Tao, and effortlessly experiencing *yangsheng* and completing the Earth Path.

- **Be open as a valley.** Open your mind, and receive happy thoughts. Open your body, and allow it to breathe and function free from conflict. Be open to your *shen* (spirit) and welcome a long and healthy life.

- **Retire when your tasks are completed.**[23] Know when to stop. Workaholics usually burn out; without health you have nothing.

- **Avoid excess, extravagance, and arrogance.**[24] Be humble and happy with the simple things in life; modesty is a virtue.

- **Those who go against The Way [of nature] come to an early end.**[25] Those who ignore the Tao and feel they know better eventually drain their life-supporting *qi*. This means that they could become sick and die prematurely if they continue to operate outside of and without the protection of the Tao.

- **Know contentment, and be rich.**[26] The principle of *yangsheng* includes striving to be contented, but not forcing it, as this is shallow and cannot be sustained. Instead, let contentment grow through subtle changes you make to your life and then experience true wealth.

- **Only those who "live out" their days have a long life.**[27] To "live out your days," you will have viewed each day with the same feeling of zest and enthusiasm, not dwelling on past days or pondering future days. Instead, you will have lived for today, and in doing so, avoided the anxiety and stress of focusing on the past and future.

- **There is no greater disaster than not being content.**[28] If you never know when enough is enough and fail to recognize when contentment is within your grasp, you will wander aimlessly, blinkered, unable to see true happiness.

- **What is firmly rooted cannot be pulled out.**[29] Those that stay grounded and patiently work their way through life's obstacles develop resilience. This combination grows strong roots in the form of mental strength (*shen*) and a stable life.

- **To forcibly add to one's natural vitality is called ill-omened.**[30] Forcing fitness through excessive exercising, thinking it is making you healthier, is now (and was also back then) believed to be counterproductive. Scientists say moderate exercise is most beneficial for health and vitality.

- **The heavy is the root of light.**[31] In this instance, "heavy" refers to someone who has discovered the Yin of the earth in their mind and body, for only when rooted, do you truly discover the lightness of Yang; in much the same way as a ball, when exposed to the power of Yin, falls to the earth (heavy), then rebounds back up (light), transformed into and embraced by Yang.

- **Shine but don't dazzle.**[32] By adjusting your lifestyle to one that balances Yin and Yang, you will stay below the radar, yet shine in any chosen path you follow. The classic Taoist way to conduct your life is to walk the earth unnoticed by the more jealous-minded in society.

# Chang San-Feng

Chang San-Feng, the creative founder of tai chi chuan, must appear in this Hall of Fame, if only because he reputedly lived to the age of 200 (mid-AD 1200–1400). Early in his life, he practiced acupuncture and qigong, but at some point rejected society, in classic Taoist tradition, and undertook a pilgrimage to the mountains to find the Truth (the meaning of life).

Here, he settled down initially to learn from Taoist recluses and then the infamous Shaolin monks. They taught him humility, patience, determination, and their much-sought-after secrets of enlightenment. After many years of contemplation and study, some say he dreamt (others say he witnessed) a white crane fighting a snake, and from their incredibly beautiful and deadly body motions created 13 Postures that would become *tai chi chuan* ("grand ultimate boxing").

His notoriety comes from the fact that he was known to have been alive during the mid-1200s and that during the 1400s, a Ming Dynasty (AD 1368–1644) emperor summoned him to court from his reclusive life in the mountains to bestow Immortal status upon him.

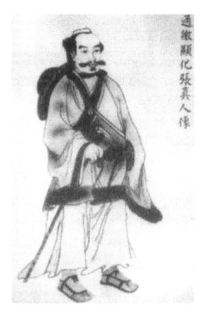

**Fig. 31** Chang San-Feng

Here are some classic longevity and enlightenment gems from the Immortal Chang:

- **Humans are the most intelligent of living beings. Because they are intelligent they should love their life.**[33] It is interesting how this corresponds with what Professor Brian Cox, renowned documentary presenter and physicist, said recently about the possibility that we could be the only sentient beings in our galaxy, and that we should do everything we can to respect and preserve what may turn out to be uniquely precious.
- **Apply your will (*shen*), not force.**[34] To pave the way to a smooth ride through life, it is wise to negotiate all obstacles in an unflustered, calm, centred, yet steadfast way (using the will/*shen*), without being drawn into frustration and anger (force).
- **There are people who are serene and free, following natural reality, whom others consider lazy, but I consider at peace.**[35] Those who follow natural reality live within the embrace of Yin and Yang, and to those whose lives fall outside they would look like they

are idling their lives away. Centred people have no need to dash about disorganized and chaotic; they always find time.

- **Unify the internal with the external.**[36] The unification of the inner (fluids and vapours) with the external (physical body) is the primary goal in tai chi and qigong training. This is when the *qi*-based energy-body (*jinglo*), the breath, and the circulatory systems unite as one system, coordinated with your physical movements.
- **Seek serenity in action.**[37] This is also known as *sung*, which is when the mind and the body are deeply relaxed, free from conflict, and able to work in unison. This is accomplished by doing less instead of more, and manifests as lightness in your step and a life naturally protected from stress and sickness.

# Li Ching Yuen

Li Ching Yuen was born in Sichuan, China, on 6 May 1677, and died aged 256 of natural causes ("died healthy") in 1933. Standing 7 feet tall, Li was a practising herbalist and a tai chi chuan, *baguazhang* (Eight Directions Palm) martial artist and qigong master. It is said that, at

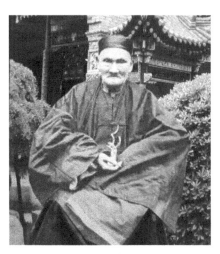

**Fig. 32** Li Ching Yuen

89

the time of his passing, he had outlived as many as 24 wives and 180 descendants. A Chinese general named Yang Sen, who had not only met him but also written an account of his long life, claimed, "He had a ruddy complexion, walked with a brisk stride, and had good eyesight and long fingernails."

The image of Li on the previous page is said to have been taken approximately six years before his death and shows his long finger nails, which are associated with longevity. There is enough factual evidence to say that, without reasonable doubt, he lived for a period of at least 200 years. (An entry in *Wikipedia* by Wu Chung-chieh, a professor at Chengdu University, asserts that Li was born in 1677, and imperial Chinese government records show that in 1827, he was formally congratulated on his 150th birthday and in 1877, on his 200th.)

It would not be unreasonable to ask, "What was he doing that enabled him to live long and die healthy?"

Well, according to one of Li's disciples, tai chi master Da Liu, his master would "perform the exercises (baguazhang, tai chi, and qigong) regularly every day, correctly and with sincerity, for a period of his life that lasted some 120 years." Li would also experiment with medicinal herbs to ward off the ravages of old age, and continued to do so throughout his life.

## The Maxims of Li Ching Yuen on How to Attain Longevity[38]

- **Every day mindful practice.** Be diligent and disciplined (without force) to practise and integrate a health-enhancing and life extending regime that suits you personally.
- **When the mind is disciplined.** Here Li refers to the *yi* mind (the wisdom mind), which controls and balances the potentially naughty twins (Yin and Yang). When disciplined, they bring harmony to your life.
- **Sleep like a dog.** Fill your days with activity so that when you retire, you naturally fall into a deep, replenishing, and relaxing sleep at the same time every night and rise at the same time every morning.

- **Walk sprightly like a pigeon.** Li is referring to walking with a brisk stride as a pigeon walks, not slouching or meandering but walking in a spirited way.
- **Sit like a tortoise.** When sitting, you should keep the hips and legs open in the lower body and the same in the arms, shoulders, and armpits in the upper body. This allows your whole body to breathe, even at rest.
- **The Way can work for us.** "The Way" is the Tao, and for the Tao to work for us, we must conduct our lives and configure our bodies and minds to allow it to flow through us.
- **Keep a quiet heart.** This overlaps with "Avoid Extremes of Emotion," as uncontrolled emotions disturb the heart. Here, Li specifically means that we should practise *jing zuo* ("sitting quietly"—see Step 6) to maintain a calm mind, heart, and spirit.
- **Sooner or later, everything comes to fruition.** Time, patience, and regular practice (*kung fu*) delivers results. If you act in accord with the Tao, your aspirations will manifest almost as a matter of course.
- **We can hold back neither the coming of flowers nor the downward rush of a stream.** Arrogant and ignorant people think that *they* know best, and they are unlikely to take well-meaning advice from others, which makes it likely that they will walk straight into disease with their eyes wide shut.

## Peng Zu (Ancestor Peng)

Living some say for a period of 800 years, throughout the Yin and Chou dynasties (1800–400 BC), Peng Zu symbolizes longevity, nutrition, and sexual therapy. His notoriety drew the attention of the kings of the Yin period, who made him a marquis of a district known as Dapeng. Peng Zu is mentioned by Confucius in *The Analects*, where he states that he is like Peng Zu, because he is a transmitter of the knowledge passed on by the ancients rather than a creator.

Peng Zu's extraordinary longevity is said to be due to the following personal hygiene disciplines:

- **Qigong:** He practised moving *qi* throughout his body with long, slow extensions of the limbs.
- **Breathing:** He combined his qigong with deep abdominal breathing.
- **Massage:** He would massage his eyes and other parts of his body with his palms.
- **Mouth Churning:** Churning his tongue around the mouth to stimulate saliva (Sweet Dew).

Peng's longevity was said to be due to his diet, qigong exercises, Taoist sexual practices, and *jing zuo*.

# Centenarians of Bama

The residents of Longevity Village[39] in Bama County in Guangxi Province have lived a charmed life that has resulted in the village gaining notoriety for having more centenarians than any other village in China. Their numbers were seven times greater than any other comparable village, and when their secret life became known, it caused quite a stir throughout China. Longevity tourism is now bringing extra income to the village, and as such, degrading all that made them special. Their once solitary and tranquil life has been lost and replaced with a tourist industry building boom.

Let's examine what life was like there prior to the village's commercialization:

## Village *Feng Shui*

Longevity Village is nestled in a valley separating two mountain ranges and has a mineral-rich, jade-coloured river running through the heart of the town. The climate is very mild, and they say that "Even in the winter, it's not cold." The air quality is very good, and the region has a strong geomagnetic field, which reputedly offers the following therapeutic benefits: regulated sleep patterns, boosted immune and nervous systems, and strong heart and brain functions.

## Diet

The villagers eat simple food centred on organic rice, green vegetables, natural oils, seldom eat meat, and drink mineral-rich water.

## Villagers' Philosophy for a Long Life

Here are the centenarians' recommendations for how to live in order to flow past 100 years:

- If you stay indoors every day, your health will decline.
- Our families care for and respect their elderly relatives.
- Be a good person.
- Have a good heart.
- Don't create unnecessary demands on yourself.
- Keep busy by working hard (farming and fishing).
- Walk a lot every day.

No doubt there are villagers who still try to live the same life as before the outside world arrived, but wealth and abundance is not always a blessing.

# Okinawa, Japan

Finally, it would be remiss in this section on long-lived people to not mention the island people of Okinawa, Japan, who through an incredibly healthy diet and great philosophy of life have become the longevity icons of modern times. They live according to the same philosophy as the Bama residents in China, but have an amazing range of healthy food at their disposal, which they embrace with gusto.

One other point: It is noticeable how the centenarians of Okinawa have incorporated "happy *qi*" into their daily lives. They work hard at enjoying life and practise laughing therapy—"Laughter is the best medicine," as the saying goes, and according to the Bible, "A cheerful heart is good medicine, but a crushed spirit dries up the bones." Once again, sadly, it is reported that their longevity island status is being eroded by the influx of Western fast-food outlets.

## Zhong-Li and Lu Discuss Longevity

**Lu:** Master, will I live longer by retreating here in the mountains with you?

**Zhong-Li:** Not necessarily. You could have lived to a ripe old age had you remained in your busy city.

**Lu:** But I thought by coming here with you I would have more chance of attaining longevity.

**Zhong-Li:** Do you think the Tao only dwells here in the mountains? The Tao is everywhere and does not weaken among the densely populated places.

**Lu:** So what is the difference between cultivating the Tao here and back in my home city?

**Zhong-Li:** In principle, there is no difference, but where many people exist you have more distractions and human-created pollution. Providing you can find a portal to serenity within the chaos, the Tao will shine through and help you live longer and die healthy.

**Lu:** Then why should I stay here, living a simple existence without the comforts afforded me at home?

**Zhong-Li:** Here, you don't have to seek a portal.

# Conclusion

What are you to take from this step? Go back and reread the information about each of the icons of longevity and contemplate their suggestions for a long, healthy life. Look at where you can make subtle changes to incorporate these into your life, and ideally, consider seeking out a qualified teacher in the Taoist arts of tai chi and qigong, who will have a much deeper understanding of their true meaning. However, there is much you can do for yourself, starting with diet, lifestyle, and exercise.

## Step 5
# Yin and Yang
# Rhythms of Life

This is where your journey along the Earth Path takes on the essential longevity rhythms that fuel your mind, body, and spirit and direct it to your destination. To do this you need to understand how these rhythms influence everything in your life, and more specifically, what they are.

Professor Carl Sagan the late, great American astronomer, astrophysicist, and cosmologist, once said: "We are the children of the cosmos, because we are made from the dust of the cosmos." If we are made from this space dust, it is reasonable to assume that the forces that influence the most distant galaxies are the same forces operating on planet Earth.

Western science would call these forces/energies gravity; electromagnetic, nuclear, and solar matter; antimatter; dark matter; and dark energy. The ancient Chinese simply called them all one name: the Tao; the active and non-active forces of the universe that represent the Tao are its children: Yin (the passive) and Yang (the active).

The earliest reference to Yin and Yang comes from the *I Ching* (*Book of Changes*), which comments on how Yin and Yang influence and drive all changes throughout the universe, from the grand to the minute.

According to the *I Ching*, a person who aligns their mind, body, and spirit with Yin and Yang becomes one of the Three Powers:

> *The sage makes good his position*
> *Between Heaven and Earth.*[40]

Yin circulates from the earth, and Yang circulates from the heavens; together, they meet in harmony in the enlightened sagelike human being, who becomes the Third Power (*tai chi*). This is only accomplished when you understand the other two powers and openly attune to them.

Aligning yourself with the rhythms and frequencies of the Tao (Yin and Yang) does not entail retreating to a mountain top and dedicating the rest of your life to growing a long white beard while sitting cross-legged in a cave (this applies to men, as well). According to Lu Dongbin:

> *Nobody wants to die. That's why followers*
> *Of the Tao cultivate to attain longevity.*[41]

## Daily *Yin* and *Yang* Life Cycle

To start this personal cultivation of attuning yourself to the Tao, it is important to live in accordance with the rhythms of the Tao. The illustration in Figure 33 shows the recommended daily life cycle of Yin and Yang that you should follow.

To understand how to live in accordance with the Yin and Yang cycle, you must sense and feel inwardly. Or, as the ancient Tao masters would say, you must "gaze inwards" at the ebb (night time) and flow (morning) of your life force, or *qi*—how tired you feel at night, and how your mind, body, and spirit gradually and naturally come to rest; how in the morning after a good night's sleep you wake up refreshed, with a mind that is sharp, a body that is energized, and a spirit that can take on all the day's challenges. According to the ancients, the Middle Path life-line must be nurtured in order to become as strong as an "eight-strand brocade," not left to become as weak as a "single strand of cotton."

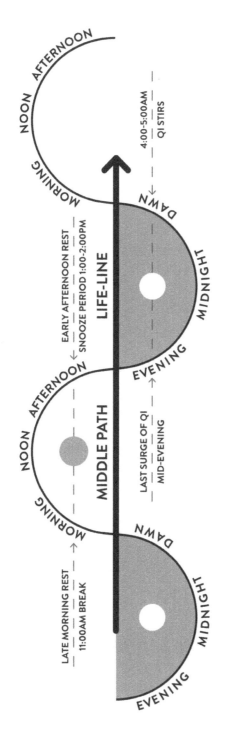

**Fig. 33** The Middle Path life cycle

Step 5

## Example of Daily *Yin* and *Yang* Life Cycle

**6 a.m.** Awaken and rise slowly; never jump out of bed. Sit on the edge of the bed, and gently perform four Crane Breathing and Spine Bowing repetitions. This will regulate your blood pressure and help prevent a drop in blood pressure upon standing. Just before you stand, lower your head and breathe out. Gradually move from sitting to standing, inhaling as you come up. Once you are fully erect, hold the in-breath for two seconds, and breathe out gently as you move away from the bed. (This is particularly beneficial for people with Parkinson's disease, hypotension disorder, COPD, and heart disease.)

**Instinct:** Need to urinate? If yes, do not delay. Remember the two Rs: Release and Replace. What leaves one end is to be replaced at the other—hydration to balance urination.

**Instinct:** Need to have a bowel movement? If yes, do not delay. Remember the principle of P & G: Perform and Go. Never sit for longer than necessary and indulge in straining, as this increases the risk of developing haemorrhoids (internal and external). These are caused by suspending the relaxed anal muscles/canal for too long, they become engorged with blood due to being gravitationally pushed downward.

**6.30 a.m.** Perform some gentle White Crane *shenkai* (stretching) and breathing movements outside in a scenic spot, facing the rising sun, followed by some or all of the Eight Daoyin.

**7.15 a.m.** Breakfast moderately.

**8 a.m.** Commence daily chores, hobbies, and other activities.

**11 a.m.** Take time out for *jing zuo* while enjoying a refreshing drink. This means just sitting quietly and not performing deep meditation. (This is represented as the small Yin in the head of Yang during the Daytime phase in the illustration.)

**12–1 p.m.** Have lunch. This is preferably the main meal of the day, as the digestive system is stronger at lunchtime than in the evening.

**1–3 p.m.** During this window, allow time for a 30–40 minute afternoon nap, or power nap, in order to boost your *qi* for the rest of the afternoon. (This is represented by the same Yin at the head of Yang during the Daytime phase.)

**5–6 p.m.** Early evening is the best time to eat a light dinner. Do not overload your digestive system when it is (like you) slowing down towards the end of a busy day.

**6–10 p.m.** Sometime during this evening window, you should feel a slight resurgence of *qi*. Use it to practise walking and standing *jing zuo*. If the weather is kind, look at the sunset and feel the earth's evening *qi*.

**10 p.m.** Time to retire to bed. Note: Two hours prior to bedtime, remove all electronic smart devices (phones, computers, tablets). Drink a small cup of chamomile tea or unsweetened or lightly sweetened hot chocolate. Create the conditions to naturally fall asleep—the perfect scenario being to arrive at the pillow with *kong* ("empty") *yi* ("a prepared, calm, and peaceful mind"). Do not take a "monkey mind" to bed with you.

**4 a.m.** Morning *qi* stirs. This is to prepare you to wake up by leading you out of a deep sleep to a lighter, shallower state, making the transition from sleep to wakefulness more natural.

**Note:** These times are not cast in stone; they are flexible to suit the individual, along with the recommended guidance that accompanies them.

# Discerning *Yin* and *Yang*

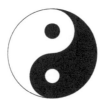

**Fig. 34** Classically depicted *Yin* and *Yang (tai chi tu)* symbol

This is how a Yin and Yang (*tai chi tu*) symbol should be depicted, with the rising Yang (white) seen above the descending Yin (black). Neither holds control of the ultimate power that is *tai chi*, the driving force of the universe; instead, they act in full mutual support of each other and are placed within each other to ensure harmony and balance. Yang becomes Yin, and Yin becomes Yang, in a never-ending cosmic dance that both creates and destroys life.

> *The myriad creatures carry on their backs the Yin*
> *And embrace in their arms the Yang,*
> *And are the blending of the generative forces of the two.*[42]

> ~ Lao Tzu

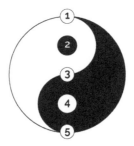

**Fig. 35** *Yin* and *Yang* key points

Within and around the symbol in Figure 35 are locations that help explain how this harmonious couple retain their equilibrium, power, and balance, seen as follows in descending order from the top of the symbol to the bottom:

1 **Small White Circle at the Top.** Maximum point of Yang, where Yang begins to transmute into Yin.
2 **Small Black Circle in the Head of Yang.** The subtle presence of Yin, its inactive anchor, stabilizing what would otherwise become a rampant Yang in a universe of chaos.
3 **Small White Circle at the Centre of the Symbol.** The Middle Path anchor and lifeline around which all things manifest in harmony.
4 **Small White Circle in the Head of Yin.** The subtle presence of Yang, its uplifting bringer of light into what would otherwise be total emptiness and darkness in a universe of chaos.
5 **Small White Circle at the Bottom.** The maximum point of Yin, where Yin begins to transmute into Yang.

In the context of health, longevity, and universally, Yin on its own means:

- **The Body Parts:** Front of torso, including the face and neck, plus the soles of the feet, palms of the hands, and inside the arms and legs, sunken chest, bent knees, head extended forwards.
- **The Body Posture:** Hollow, sunken chest; bent knees; chin and head extended forward; coccyx tilted under (inwards).
- **The Body Function:** Breathing out, digestion, defecation, white-coloured urination, sleeping, meditation, sighing, and anaemia.
- **Emotions:** Grief, depression, craving, obsession, hatred, jealousy, negative thinking.
- **Direction of Motion:** Down, back, sinking, contraction, and inward.
- **Body Conditions:** Hypotension (low blood pressure), anaemia, cancer, hypothermia.

- **Generally:** Night time, moon, space, black holes, earth, eye of the storm, oceans, lakes, rivers, streams, waterfalls, rain, snow, low pressure weather, women, children, internet, peace.

In the context of health, longevity, and universally, Yang on its own means:

- **The Body:** Back of the torso, forehead, and top and back of head, outside of the arms, hands, and legs.
- **The Body Posture:** Pigeon chest (pushed out); straight, locked back of the knees; chin excessively tucked inwards; neck joints locked straight; coccyx tilted outwards.
- **The Body Function:** Breathing in, indigestion (reflux), constipation, dark orange urination, awake, and shouting.
- **Emotions:** Happiness, contentment, love, positive thinking, anger, over-thinking.
- **Direction of Motion:** Up, forward, floating, expansion, and outward.
- **Body Condition:** Hypertension (high blood pressure), stroke, dermatitis, hyperthermia.
- **Generally:** Daytime, sun, white holes in space (still theoretical), sky, storms, mountains, volcanoes, hail, high pressure weather, men, the elderly, and wars.

This list of things Yin or Yang is just a minute example. In fact, Yin and Yang encompass everything in the known universe and are superbly portrayed in Figure 36, where Earth is clearly split between day (Yang white) and night (Yin black) and spins on its axis over a 24-hour period (the imaginary line between the black spot in Yang and the white spot in Yin). Here, Yin and Yang are in harmony, which creates balance; through this balance, life begins, life extends, life ends.

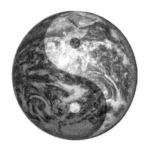

**Fig. 36** *Yin* and *Yang* on Earth

From out of chaos, peace and harmony appear. To this day, the universe demonstrates how this works:

- **Grand Scale Yang:** The explosive and chaotic beginnings of life in the universe are supernova events and the unimaginable forces at work in the birth of stars.
- **Grand Scale Yin:** In the incalculable expanse of space, where nothing exists but stillness and emptiness, is dark matter, the invisible hands pulling the galaxies together, and dark energy, its invisible counter-balance.
- **Extreme Yang:** The most powerful Yang forces in the universe are gamma-ray bursts. They dwarf the supernova events, and are an unbelievable million, trillion times brighter than our sun.
- **Extreme Yin:** Appearing in various grades of vastness, the ultimate Yin force in the universe must be the all-consuming black hole.

## Sensing and Feeling *Yin* and *Yang*

Academically knowing how, when, and where Yin and Yang forces appear and interface with one another is not enough. As my revered teacher, Grandmaster Dr. Yang, Jwing-Ming, explains, "Knowing is not enough; you must feel their presence in action throughout your body and mind." This is also described as "becoming *tai chi*."

The following actions may help guide you:

- **Breathe in as you stand up after sitting:** Using the correct body mechanics (See *San Tsai,* Step 8) start breathing in (through the nose) just before you push upwards from your feet, and sense the whole body being inflated with air and driven upwards. This is Yang.
- **Breathe out as you sit down after standing:** Using the same principle, breathe out slowly as you naturally lower your body into the sitting position. The out-breath should be released as if it is the air itself that is lowering you. This is Yin.
- **Breathe in as you lift your arms:** In order to lift your arms correctly, the power for the lift must commence in the feet and travel up the legs through the centre of the torso (just in front of the spine), which will naturally elevate the chest and head. Swing the elbows outwards, and observe the arms lift effortlessly. This is Yang.
- **Breathe out as you lower the arms:** Consciously relax your knees forward, start breathing out, and feel the pelvis sink, followed by the chest and head. Then bend the elbows to make them point down, and allow the arms to lower, as if controlled by the slow releasing of the breath. This is Yin.
- **Breathe in as you turn the head, torso, and waist to look behind:** Again, the impetus must start in the feet to lift the torso and head while turning the waist and head to gaze behind. This is Yang.
- **Breathe out as you return to face front:** Return your head to face front slowly and gently, while still holding the breath in, and just as the head arrives in the forward-facing position, slowly release the breath as your waist, chest, and shoulders follow the head to face front. This is Yin.
- **Breathe in as you pull towards you:** Any pulling action from any direction should be applied from the feet and appear in the upper body as a lifted chest and head with elbows bending and pointing outwards. This is Yang, because the object or person you are pulling is being projected toward you.
- **Breathe out as you push away:** Concentrating the push to the outside edge of the hands creates more focused power at the point

of contact. As you release the push, lower the abdomen, chest, and shoulders as you extend the arms to push the object away. This is Yin.

- **Breathe in as you lift the heels:** This applies to stretching/reaching upwards as you breathe in, and opens all of the extending muscles of the body. This is Yang.
- **Breathe out as you lower your heels to the ground:** This applies to lowering the stretched body back to earth; if continued, full squatting on the earth will occur. This is Yin.

## Yang Posture

The posture demonstrated in Figure 37 is known as Heaven Posture and is the highest of the classical postures contained within the arts of tai chi and qigong. Holding this posture for a short period (2 minutes) will connect you to Heavenly *qi*, which when absorbed:

- Lifts your mood.
- Increases your body energy throughout.
- Makes you feel physically light and vibrant.
- Boosts the energy in the brain.

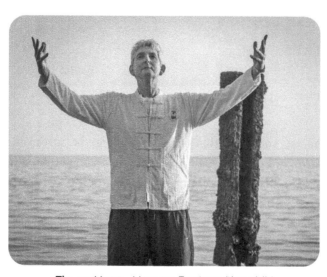

**Fig. 37** *Yang*—Heaven Posture *(tien shih)*

## Yin Posture

The posture demonstrated in Figure 38 is known as Earthing Posture and is the foundation of the classical postures contained within the arts of tai chi and qigong. Holding this posture for a couple of minutes will connect you to Earth *qi,* which, when absorbed:

- Calms the "monkey mind," which chatters incessantly.
- Stabilizes your body, lowering the risk of falls, and improves athletic performance.
- Roots the body and mind, strengthening the *shen* ("spirit").
- Helps control tremors in Parkinson's disease.
- Drains the strength out of panic attacks and anxiety.

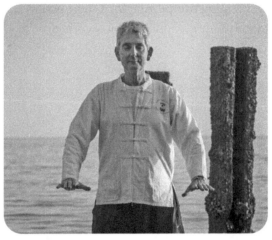

**Fig. 38** *Yin—Earthing Posture (jiedi shih)*

As you can see, the separation of the two energy postures can be positive to health and general wellbeing, but when you combine them in a flowing sequence intimately linked to your natural nose breathing, you create balance. To perform the postures, you should:

- Stand with your feet shoulder-width apart, with feet pointing forward and arms hanging at the side.
- Keep the head erect, with eyes on the distant horizon.

- Strike the pose shown in Figure 10, rest the eyelids, and breathe gently in and out three times.
- Open the eyes, and tilt the head up, as if gazing at the moon, while gradually breathing in.
- Raise the centre of the chest, and allow both arms to naturally float upward to strike the pose seen in Figure 37 (still breathing in).
- Lower the head, eyes, chest, and arms to return to Figure 38 (Earthing Posture), while gradually breathing out.
- Repeat the whole sequence four times.

This routine is called *tien–kun qigong*, which means "Heaven and Earth Energy/Breathing Training." It is a classic example of the "dual cultivation" of *qi* throughout the body, as explained by tai chi and qigong grandmaster Dr. Yang, Jwing-Ming:

> *If you understand how* qi *functions and*
> *Know how to regulate it correctly,*
> *You should be able to live a long and healthy life.*[43]

## Zhong–Li and Lu Discuss Yin and Yang

**Lu:** Master, when you say we are all children of the Tao, what do you mean?

**Zhong-Li:** The Tao is the primordial source from where our universe was born, and at this stage chaos existed, from which harmony would eventually emerge. To create this harmony, the Tao had to move among all things, including human life, and took the form of *tai chi*, the Supreme Ultimate Force.

**Lu:** Is tai chi, therefore, another name for the Tao?

**Zhong-Li:** Yes, the Tao is tai chi, which is the parent of Yin and Yang, and to spread its influence throughout all things, it split into two polar opposites of itself. These opposites are the children of the Tao; one was named Yin and the other Yang. Yin represents feminine, darkness, earth, stability, decline, and death, while Yang represents masculine, light, space, growth, and life. Just like children lacking the influence of a parent, they can become unruly and chaos could return. To prevent this, tai chi was created to be such a parent, whose role is to constantly keep the children in perfect harmony.

**Lu:** So, as we are the universe, Yin and Yang, I must assume, resides within?

**Zhong-Li:** We are not exempt from the Supreme Ultimate Force; as it breathes its influence through all things, we also feel its breath, for we are a microcosmic version of the living universe, and what happens on a macrocosmic scale also happens to us. Those who understand this and conduct their lives according to the rhythms of Yin and Yang are able to fulfil the allotted period of life that the Tao bestows upon us.

**Lu:** But what of those who die early?

**Zhong-Li:** Some die through wars or accidents and disease, while others die prematurely because they know nothing of Yin and Yang. Some knowingly walk a different path, and by doing so, lose the protection that Yin and Yang afford. This results in a chaotic life, often cut short.

**Lu:** So, the Tao flows through us via Heaven and Earth, both of which provide the rhythms for health and happiness in our daily lives. These rhythms, I assume, are Yin *qi* and Yang *qi*, both of which provide the guidance, insights, and momentum for our longevity?

**Zhong-Li:** Yes.

# Spirit Guide Reveal

In the early 1980s, during sleep, I saw a bearded man standing before me in traditional Chinese clothing, and to his left-hand side, hovering in mid-air, was the tai chi symbol.

I asked him who he was.

He replied, "I am the one who will show you your life path."

And then he pointed to the symbol, specifically the Yin sector, and said, "This is you. You will bring light into the lives of those lost in the dark."

He was, in fact, pointing directly at the small white circle of Yang embedded in the head of Yin. At the time, I knew that this was significant, but I did not realize how significant until some years later, when I was employed by Warner Leisure, a national hotel and leisure group, to teach at one of their holiday retreats in North Wales, a No Children Allowed holiday centre that attracted guests from all over the UK and beyond.

This was at a time when tai chi and qigong were generally unknown to the public, so when I stood on stage in their theatre, which housed up to 200 guests, and shared the physical and philosophical gems of tai chi and qigong, their response (every week) was what the spirit guide had suggested. In the main, they were astounded by the immediate beneficial impact on them physically and mentally—out of the dark and into the light.

# Conclusion

This step has hopefully helped you understand the basic concept of Yin and Yang and how these two precious gems can greatly improve the quality of your life, setting you firmly on the path of health and longevity. The next step dovetails with this one and builds on all previous steps, as you enter the realm of *neigong* ("inner gazing"). To help put this step into perspective, based on the conversation between Zhong-Li and Lu above, the following interrelationship structure should be of some use:

Tai Chi = Wisdom Mind
Wisdom Mind = Yin and Yang Balance
Yin and Yang Balance = Life Balance

# Step 6
# *Jing Zuo*—How to Sit Quietly

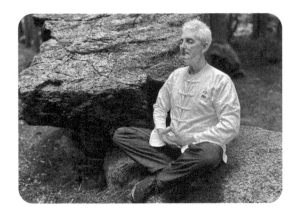

At some time in their lives, most people living in our modern era will be exposed to pressures and demands similar to those that affected people living thousands of years ago. These include work pressures, caring for the family, famine, wars and forced flight, to name but a few.

All were, and still are, experiences that switch on the sympathetic nervous system (fight-or-flight) in the body. If, as is often the case, sympathetic arousal is sustained over a long period of time, it puts a strain on vital neurochemicals in the brain. This results in symptoms such as anxiety, fatigue, loss of appetite, suppressed immunity, memory loss, confusion, depression, and insomnia.

According to the ancient Chinese, these conditions, if left unchecked, give rise to the "monkey mind" (mental chatter) that emanates from the cerebral cortex of the brain. The ancients found that *jing zuo* ("sitting quietly") would calm down the monkeys and combat this common mental health issue. In modern times, we would recognize this as meditation. If practised regularly, *jing zuo* not only removes the chatter but opens doors to new and interesting realms.

In Step 6, you will be introduced to *jing zuo* and take your first steps into the fascinating world of "inner gazing" and "stillness" training. There are a variety of meditation practices, some of which can be quite sophisticated and difficult to master without the express guidance of a qualified teacher. Here, however, we will be applying *jing zuo* in its simplest form, which just so happens to be the best form.

Notably, this step comes just before Step 7, where you will commence *shen* ("spirit") training, where it is said:

> *To nourish the* shen *("spirit"), you must first control human passion, eliminate monkey emotions, still the mind, and practise long breathing.*
>
> ~ Taoist teaching

## The *Jing Zuo* Perspective

To "sit quietly" does not necessarily mean on the floor with your legs tied uncomfortably in knots. It refers to sitting anywhere and on anything (see Figure 39).

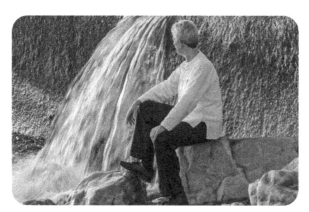

**Fig. 39** *Jing Zuo*—Sitting Quietly

Sitting quietly by a waterfall in the fresh morning air and incorporating the posture advice given in Step 2 will settle both mind and body. *Jing zuo*, therefore, must be mutually supported by good posture and natural "long breathing," which explains why this step follows steps 2 and 3, specifically.

As alluded to earlier, *jing zuo* also translates to mean "meditation," and "medi" means "middle" or "centre"; therefore, by "sitting quietly," you guide yourself onto the Middle Path, where you will find your true centre. People who are "centred" are embracing the powerful Middle Path lifeline (see Figure 33).

*Jing zuo* on its own is not enough. All three tangible (structural) and non-tangible (etheric) things that make us human—mind, body, and spirit—must be equally nurtured, which is why we have the three Paths of Zhong-Li and Lu. The Earth Path guidance in this book is meant to physically nurture the body, calm the mind, and stir the spirit in preparation for Middle Path exploration. Without the nurtured physical body, the mind cannot be stilled, and without a stilled mind, the spirit is not stirred. *Jing zuo* is the essential link and facilitator between body and spirit.

## Reasons to Practise *Jing Zuo* Meditation

- **To Regulate the Mind:** To recapture the mind's untainted purity and maintain an empty mind free from conflict.
- **For Mental Health:** To centre the mind (*yi*), to clear the senses, and find the place where you can see and feel everything within and around you. This is accomplished through daily practice of *Jing Zuo*.
- **For Physical Health and Self-Healing:** The human body (*ren ti*) functions best when the mind and body are calm, allowing it to switch on its inner healing and balancing processes. The ancients maintained that *jing zuo* can cure one hundred illnesses.
- **To Improve Physical and Mental Performance:** Your strength of spirit (*shen*) plays a major role in accomplishing goals and overcoming challenges. *Jing zuo* fuels and frees your *shen* and allows you to keep going when things get tough.

- **To Regulate the Breathing**: Your life force (*qi*) is fuelled by the breath, and optimum breathing is assisted by a calm, centred, and focused mind, and this is only made possible by developing the mind of a sage.
- **To Regulate Life:** *Yangsheng* describes the much-sought-after goals in life. By helping you maintain a regular Yin and Yang life cycle, *jing zuo* can guide you along the Earth Path with vision and clarity.

Generally, *jing zuo* is used to clear mental space and allow the mind to experience peaceful contemplation and unrestricted potential.

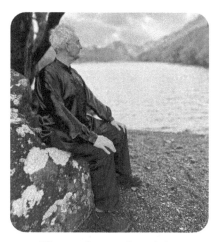

**Fig. 40** *Jing zuo* by a lake

## How to Practise *Jing Zuo*

Good *jing zuo* practice starts with precautionary notes in the form of do's and don'ts. Here are a few to consider:

- **DO** practice daily, but not in excess; 10 minutes is adequate for beginners. At the same time, do not fret if, due to unplanned distractions or demands, you miss your session. You will soon discover that *jing zuo* can be practised anywhere at any time.
- **DO NOT** practise *jing zuo* while under the influence of drugs or alcohol, as this will do more damage than good. A mind that is

intoxicated by chemicals will resist the Tao's ability to calm and centre and may also manifest as mood swings.

- **DO** allow at least one hour to elapse after eating before you commence "sitting quietly." The mind state and the digestive system are sensitively linked, so while undigested food sits in the gut, the mind is subconsciously busy assisting digestion.
- **DO NOT** practice *jing zuo* when exhausted as this can tip over into instant sleep, which, as mentioned earlier, is totally different from meditation and has a totally different outcome.
- **DO** shower or bathe before commencing in order to create a relaxed body and mind. The shower or bath should be warm, neither too hot nor too cold, as these conditions can affect your *qi* by increasing or reducing its flow, respectively.
- **DO NOT** practise *jing zuo* outdoors under extreme climatic conditions, such as direct sunlight, wind, rain, humidity, cold, and damp. In much the same way as bathing in water that is too hot or too cold can negatively affect your *qi*, climatic extremes can cause negative feng shui.
- **DO** use your best instincts to choose where to practise, favouring an atmosphere and location that is tranquil, safe, and quiet that has good *qi*, which is associated with positive feng shui.
- **DO NOT** wear tight-fitting clothing or underwear, as your body needs to be free to breathe. The location of your waistband is especially important, as it is where your *zhen dan tien* ("real field of energy") resides. Any restriction around this area blocks the free passage of *qi* that flows in and out with every breath you take (I feel a song coming on).
- **DO** visit the toilet before *jing zuo* practice. It was interesting to hear a doctor specializing in sexual health say recently that it is better to empty the bowels and the bladder before making love, as this will improve the experience. In a strange and obtuse way, *jing zuo* is also more pleasurable and beneficial when you have had a "clearout," because there is nothing in the pelvic basin to cause *qi* blockage.
- **DO NOT** attempt to practise *jing zuo* if you are experiencing chronic hyper- or hypotension, or any other illness that impacts your health,

without discussing it first with a medical professional and qualified tai chi/qigong instructor. *Jing zuo* is perfectly safe and positively therapeutic when practised using the correct posture and breathing.

- **DO** gently massage the whole body, from head to toe, at the end of each session, as this will gently encourage your circulation to fire back up. Remember: If you have been sitting with legs folded, slowly straighten them out while massaging them.
- **DO NOT** practise deep, long, abdominal breathing or over-concentration on the lower abdomen while menstruating or pregnant. Just sitting quietly and breathing gently through the nose is preferred, and is still beneficial in this instance.
- **DO NOT** attempt *jing zuo* while emotionally charged. Wait a while for your mind to settle, then sit quietly with no thoughts, no expectations, and just witness the arrival of blissful stillness.

This list is for guidance only and should be reinforced with a large portion of common sense.

Dr. Jou, Tsung-Hwa, a great and much-missed tai chi master, made these comments about how to approach training with *jing zuo*:[44]

- *Jing zuo* means sitting still with a peaceful mind.
- We can look forward to meditation (*jing zuo*) as if it were a vacation.
- With a mind wide open as a valley, meditate (*jing zuo*) diligently, and allow experience to show what is true.

## Alternative Stand Still Meditation

It is not necessary to only practise sitting *jing zuo*; standing is also a viable option, and in fact, it is advisable to mix the two. This method is also known as Stand Still Posture, and is described in the *I Ching,* China's ancient book on divination. In Taoist circles, it is often called *Tao Shih,* or the Natural Way Posture. In the Western world, physiotherapists call it Standing Release Posture, as it returns the body to its default programme (natural repose), where the functioning energy, physiology, structures, and mental processes all rebalance and centre themselves.

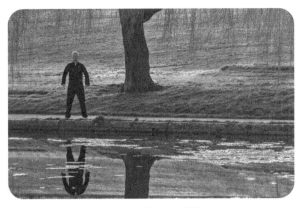

**Fig. 41** Outdoors Stand Still—*Jing Zuo*

To establish a Stand Still Posture you should loosen the whole body slowly, typically with *Daoyin* No. 1 (described in Step 8), following the instructions given. Then stand with the feet shoulder-width apart, toes pointing forward. Strike the posture seen earlier in Figure 10, with the chest slightly raised to centre the torso. Naturally open the armpits, and relax and centre the knees. The crown of the head must be raised directly upward with the chin gently tucked, in order to gravitationally centre the whole body.

The combination of sitting and standing establishes the "home centre." Gravity threads its way through the physical body, along with the mind and the spirit through

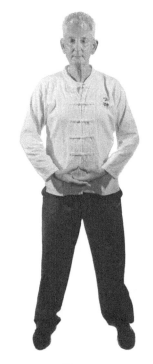

**Fig. 42**
Holding the Centre—*Jing Zuo*

stillness, and this is where it returns home. Holding this centre, with the hands positioned and shaped as shown in Figure 42, concentrates the mind, and therefore, the *qi* at the "real centre—the field of energy" (*zhen zhong—dan tien*).

The exact location of the "real centre" is shown in Figure 44. It is where the mind should rest awhile when practising *jing zuo*. Once this has been re-established the body has a central reference point that maintains natural balance, whether the body is in motion or in stillness. This has a major impact on the maintenance and enhancement of your health, and is fundamental to any aspiration to live long and die healthy.

## Guidance on Sitting or Standing Meditation

1  After sitting or standing comfortably, you should rest the eyelids but not close them. Leaving the eyes fully open distracts the mind, while closing the eyes fully is forced and therefore, unnatural.

2  Regulate your breathing through the nose to establish long, profound breathing. This refers to "long" as regards the time it takes to inhale and exhale, and "long" as regards how the breath should be sensed, descending deep down into the lower abdomen.

3  As you breathe in, imagine that the whole body is being gently illuminated with light. This type of visualization helps clear the pathways so that the *qi* can both fill and empty from the body.

4  As you breathe out, imagine your whole body is *fang sung*, relaxing and releasing. Visualizing this effect helps you deeply connect with the soft tissues, a prerequisite for *ti huxi* ("whole body breathing").

5  Feel for the Three Essential Mechanics of Breathing (see Figure 16, plus notes). Remember to sense the mechanics and avoid being driven by intention or instruction. Simply witness the Tao as it does it for you.

6  Place the tip of your tongue lightly on the roof of the mouth behind the two front teeth. This creates the bridge between two major energy meridians by completing the Small Heavenly Cycle, which comprises the Governor (*Du*) and Conception (*Ren*) meridians. The Small

Heavenly Cycle runs up the spine, starting at the centre of the pelvic floor (*huiyin*) where the Du meridian begins, over the head, down the front of the body, and under the pelvic floor, returning to the *huiyin* point where the Ren meridian ends. The place where the tongue touches is called the Yin and Yang Magpie Bridge, and is where both meridians meet in the top half of the body. By placing your tongue in this position, you strengthen the bond between them (see Figure 44, Small Heavenly Cycle—Step 7).

7  The "sweet dew" saliva will accumulate; swallow, and breathe out, allowing the *qi* to sink to the *zhen dan tien*. It also carries digestive enzymes that assist the digestive system.

8  Lightly touch the top and bottom front teeth together leaving space for the tongue to rest. This also creates the space for the sweet dew to pool before you swallow it. By consciously touching the teeth together, you prevent the mouth from dropping open.

9  Let the mind settle on its own without interference from you. This is the principle of *wuwei*, which translates to mean "do nothing"; through this non-doing, you free the Tao to guide you to *sung* ("deep relaxation").

10  Become conscious of the soft sound of your breathing, and smile. Listening quietly to your breathing has the same effect as listening to the gentle sound of the waves lapping on a beach to still the mind. Smiling helps release calming endorphins, such as serotonin, and fools your brain into thinking you are happy.

11  Allow yourself to drift to a heightened state of awareness while remaining deeply relaxed. This heightened state does not mean that your conscious mind is switched on, like a radar scanning everything around you; to the contrary, a still mind allows your hearing and psychic perception to operate in perfect clarity, both internally and externally.

12  Stay in this special place for a few minutes, gradually increasing the time spent as you practise further. With regular practice and determination (*kung fu*), you will be able to envelop yourself in the shield of stillness found in this *jing zuo* special place at will— anytime, anyplace, anywhere.

## *Jing Zuo* Special Place

The inner process of *jing zuo* guides your mind to a place that can be only described as a peaceful void, an inner haven, where all thoughts melt away, leaving you with a pure sense of just "being." It is a place that only materializes when the Yin and Yang minds cease to dance around and with each other. The special place where they merge is known in Taoist circles as *wuji* and can be likened to the stillness present in the eye of a storm, a place where profound breathing resides, patiently waiting for our homecoming. When you arrive home, as the result of time, patience and discovery, you can whisper in thankful tones, *"Huanying hui jia"* ("Welcome, home").

## Brain Wave Function

- **Alpha Waves:** Alpha waves are the brain's normal and healthy functioning state. They benefit mood as they release the brain chemical serotonin, which calms the nervous system and lowers blood pressure and heart rate and the production of stress hormones. *Jing zuo* is known to strengthen Alpha waves.
- **Beta Waves:** A joint research study into Beta waves carried out by Sydney University, Australia and the Norwegian University of Science and Technology (NTNU) in March 2010 found that they showed little to no increase in activity during *jing zuo*.[45] Beta waves are associated with a brain that is strongly engaged in debate and conversation. They switch the brain to reasoning and responding, especially during tasks involving deep thought and focused attention.
- **Theta Waves:** The same study indicated that during *jing zuo,* Theta waves increase in the frontal part of the brain, which allows us to monitor our inner experiences. This matches perfectly with the Taoist concept of "gazing inwards."
- **Delta Waves:** Delta waves are normally associated with the sleep state. They do not dominate during *jing zuo*, however, which scientists confirm. There is a difference between meditation and sleep.

The conclusion from the above findings, therefore, is that *jing zuo* appears to encourage relaxing, Alpha-wave *sung* conditions, and relaxed Theta-wave "inner gazing" to help direct our inner awareness of the mind and its activity during meditation.

## Zhong-Li and Lu Discuss Jing Zuo

**Lu:** Master, I now know that we are Yin and Yang, but how do we sense, feel, and strengthen their rhythms within us?

**Zhong-Li:** You have to understand how they ebb and flow, both internally and externally. To experience this, you must gaze inward.

**Lu:** How can I gaze inward when I can only see outward?

**Zhong-Li:** To gaze inward you must use the mind's eye, not your real eyes.

**Lu:** And how do I connect to my mind's eye?

**Zhong-Li:** By *jing zuo* ("sitting quietly"), resting your eyelids on your real eyes, and opening your mind and body to see and feel their subtle interaction within.

**Lu:** When I sit quietly I sometimes feel drowsy and wish to sleep. What is the difference between *jing zuo* and sleeping?

**Zhong-Li:** When you are asleep, so too are your mind and body, as both enter a deep state of Yin. But when you practise *jing zuo*, your mind and body are still awake in a state of pure consciousness called *wuji*. This is a place of perfect clarity, where the mind and body become centred—where stillness (*jijing*) manifests.

**Lu:** And what does stillness offer us?

**Zhong-Li:** A radiant spirit.

**Lu:** How can I see a radiant spirit?

**Zhong-Li:** Look at me.

# Conclusion

Diligent practice must not feel like a burden. You should gently introduce this discipline into your daily life and greet it like a long-lost friend.
You are now granted the ability to control your stress and anxiety from
within, where your "wisdom mind" (*chih*) establishes itself to protect
you from yourself.

*The Old Master (Lao Tzu) is said to prescribe*
*methodical calmness* (jing zuo),
*which is undeniably one of the major ingredients*
*in life-prolonging recipes and exercises by Taoists.*[46]

# Step 7
# Stirring the *Shen*—
# The Hidden Taoist Secret

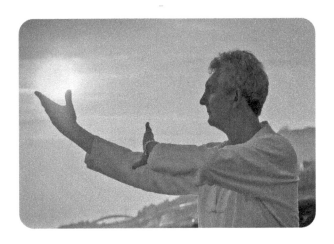

*Shen* translates to "spirit" and is one of the three human treasures of *nei dan* ("internal alchemy"); the other two being *ching* and *qi*. Basically, *ching* is the original essence inherited from your parents and established within so that you can continue the cycle and pass it down to your own children. Known as "coarse *qi*," it stems from the kidneys and manifests in the seeds of life for men and women to create human life.

The alchemical processes involved in the interactions among *ching*, *qi*, and *shen* are too complicated for the Earth Path, so you will only be introduced here to the primordial *shen*, which we are born with and that drives us on our journey through life.

As explained earlier, *kung fu* refers to the effort and determination maintained over time to achieve whatever your goals may be in life, and is usually associated with Chinese martial arts. This *shen* vapour (*ling qi*) is supportive at rest, irresistible when focused, and is the human manifestation of *Yang qi*, the expansive energetic force that must be kept under control.

Shen *is the hidden vapour within* kung fu.

~ Sifu

Ancestor Lu helps us understand *shen* through the following description:

*In humans, it is the spirit, the light in the eyes, thought in the mind;*
*it is wisdom and intelligence, innate knowledge, and capacity;*
*it is the government of vitality and energy, awareness, and understanding;*
*it is the basis of the physical shell and foundation of the life span.*[47]

*Shen* can be seen as our willpower, resolve, purpose, fortitude, determination, strength of mind, and character. It radiates outwards when we need to enforce ourselves, and inwards when we need to be more conciliatory, and providing we remain mentally and physically balanced, both are equally strong.

## *Shen,* the Root of Human Life

*Shen* is said to reside in the heart and travels through the body via the *zhong mai*, which coincides with the "gravitational centre line" that runs from the crown of the head to the centre of the pelvic floor (see Figure 44, points 1 to 2). The *zhong mai* is like a lift shaft that runs through the centre of a high-rise building with *shen* servicing all floors. For the *shen* to continue to support us in life, we must ensure that the "lift shaft" remains clear of debris and structurally aligned. In Figure 43, the *shen* "lift shaft" connects the three major energy centres of the body, identified as locations 3, 4, and 5.

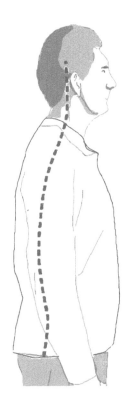

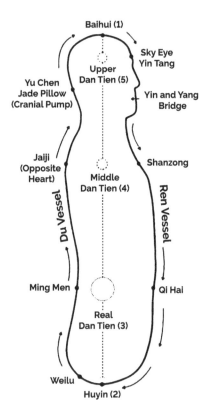

**Fig. 43** *Zhong mai—*
the central energy channel

**Fig. 44** *Xiao Zhou Tien—*
Small Heavenly Cycle

The *zhong mai* seen in Figure 43 is the home and conduit of the *shen*, which, in this image, shows a more realistic view, as it follows the natural contours of the body vertically. For the *shen* to radiate naturally throughout the body, sustained upright posture is essential. Only then can the "lift shaft" allow free passage for the *shen* to travel. The ability to maintain a "*shen* mind" (also known as "wisdom mind") is the key to a positive, confident, and healthy person.

The arrows circling the torso in Figure 44 indicate the directional flow of the Small Heavenly Cycle (SHC), or *Xiao Zhou Tien*, also known as the Microcosmic Orbit. It is a vital energy (*qi*) circuit that usually flows unabated, but can weaken if your Yin and Yang lose their equilibrium. The circuit has been designed to service organs with *qi*. The Yang organs receive *qi* from the *Du* meridian and the Yin organs from the *Ren* meridian. Chinese medicine states: "When the SHC [Small Heavenly Cycle] is full, the *shen* becomes centred and radiates throughout the body, warding off 100 illnesses."

*Shen* is also responsible for stabilizing and centring the mind, for when a mind is centred it becomes wise and is free from the extremes of emotions.

> *It is the "wisdom mind" (yi) that creates*
> *the conditions for the* shen *to be raised.*
>
> ~ Sifu

Taoists say, "There is *shen* in every human." They also say, "*Shen* is so mysterious that words limit, because the infinite Tao is limitless." Within all of us lies a mystery, and according to Taoist belief, it is the mystery of all mysteries. To negotiate the Earth Path, you only need to work on creating the conditions for your *shen* to be free. When you can maintain these conditions, you will be ready to walk the Middle Path.

> *When* shen *fills you, all six senses become clear.*
>
> ~ Sifu

## Seeing and Sensing *Shen*

Where is the *shen*? How do you find it? Well, the answers lie in the words of the ancient sages:

> Shen *shines with the brilliance of a 1,000 suns,*
> *And yet an unguided human will suppress its light.*
>
> ~ Taoist teaching

The naturally occurring light that is *shen* will surface and radiate in people who are happy, healthy (mentally and physically), and contented. It shines throughout good posture and dims when your posture loses its structure, as seen in Figures 45 and 46, which illustrate how *shen* can be limited to just below the surface (Figure 45—weak *shen*) or radiate upward and outward, filling your posture and mind positively (Figure 46—strong *shen*).

Of course, you do not need to strike a pose to switch on *shen*; you can simply "sit quietly" with the mind "empty and still," as illustrated in Figures 39 and 40. In this way, the *shen* glows gently rather than dazzling in a more animated posture and activated, driven mind.

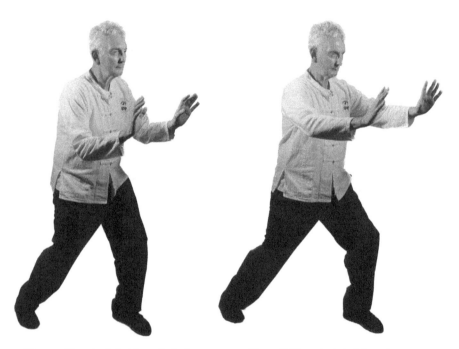

**Fig. 45** Classic *tai chi* push *(tui)*— weak *shen*

**Fig. 46** Classic *tai chi* push— strong *shen*

*Shen* is not limited to humans and can be seen in all creatures on the earth, such as the solitary heron (see Figure 47).

*Shen* manifests in the heron through its patience and focus when poised silently in perfect stillness waiting for its next meal to materialize. This represents the most natural vision of *shen*, untainted, part of the fabric of nature, directing all thoughts, instincts, and actions. We humans are no exception, in that *shen* naturally occurs within, inspiring us in just the same way, unless we impose restrictions on its functioning.

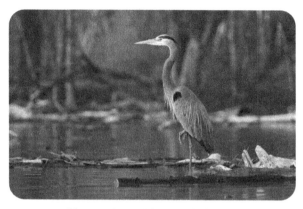

**Fig. 47** The spirit of a still heron

If you conduct your life understanding how to *see shen* in yourself and others, you should be able to note the following when it breaks the surface: a refreshed, healthy complexion; clear, sparkling eyes; lustrous hair; and a voice that sounds as clear as a bell. When you *feel shen*, this will exhibit as a sense of warmth, fullness, and vitality throughout the body; a happy, optimistic outlook; and a noticeable drop in contracting colds and viruses.

The Earth Path expects no more than this, and if you accomplish *seeing* and *feeling shen* to the level described above, you can expect to sustain a normal, long, and healthy life.

> *In ancient times, those who understood the Tao patterned themselves upon Yin and Yang and lived in harmony with the arts of divination. There was temperance of eating and drinking, Their hours of rising and retiring were regular, and not disorderly and wild. By these means, the ancients kept their bodies united with their souls, so as to fulfil their allotted lifespan completely, measuring unto a hundred years before passing away [dying healthy].*[48]

> ~ Nei Ching

# *Shen* and Health

*Shen* is of great importance in promoting human health and evolution because:

- *Shen* governs the life-maintaining functions of the body.
- It is the master of humankind.
- It is known as the "Iron Guardian" (Guardian *qi*).
- Its origin comes from stillness.
- Its existence is intimately connected with the human body.
- It naturally gravitates towards purity, and only the mind can disturb it.

*Shen* and health are intrinsically linked, and in TCM (Traditional Chinese Medicine), it is said that:

> Shen *and the Guardian* qi *(immune system and external* qi *field that envelopes and protects the body) operate as one.*

When the *shen* is weak, so is the body energy field and immune system. Tai chi and qigong switch over the brain and central nervous system to the mode of operation in which the neurotransmitters responsible for activating the immune system are produced. And let us not forget, tai chi and qigong are the earthly instruments of the Tao, and when both of these "instruments" are played skilfully and purely, beautiful music (*shen*) appears.

> *Tai chi guides us to our "centre"* (shen *residence).*
> *And qigong heals us on the way.*
>
> ~ Sifu

The important thing you must grasp is to let your inner light (*shen*) shine through. Did you notice that you were requested to *let* and not *make* your body radiate health from within? You must create the conditions for the *shen* to naturally switch on.

# Spirit Guide Reveal

*Before me stands a human form that raises its arms and spreads them apart at shoulder height, with open palms facing outwards. The figure's opaque body slowly becomes radiant, lighting up its organs, blood vessels, muscles, sinews, and nerve pathways, and still its brilliance increases until eventually, it becomes completely transparent (like a rainbow). Finally, the immense glow of a thousand suns makes me avert my gaze. Then, as if the point had been made, everything returns gradually to normal.*

This gem of an insight kindly presented by heavenly guides contains such simplicity in its message, and yet, is profound in suggesting how limitless powers of the universe await those who align with the vapours of the Tao.

To complete the Earth stage, you will need to perform *San Tsai* ("Three Powers") illustrated in the following Step 8, especially when you realize that the three powers are: Heaven, Earth, and an enlightened human being. The controlling factor of attuning yourself to the Yin of Earth and the Yang of Heaven is to centre and stabilize the *shen*. One final point to consider is:

Shen *is not* Yin, *and* shen *is not* Yang.
*It is the constant light that shines through
and helps stabilize both, and is the intimate link
to the wisdom minds in all humans.*

~ Sifu

Shen therefore should be seen as the inner force that holds us together physically, emotionally, and spiritually. Its potential is immeasurable and its source unfathomable. It is pure Dao radiating throughout the human form, without which achieving our longevity goals would remain purely an aspiration. So, hold this precious gift close to your heart for this is where it resides.

## Zhong-Li and Lu Discuss *Shen*

**Lu:** Master, what is *shen*, and where does it reside?

**Zhong-Li:** *Shen* is a highly refined form of *qi* and is the most powerful force within you. It resides in your heart but manifests through the central core of your mind and body.

**Lu:** Does *shen* in any way rely on a constant supply of *qi?*

**Zhong-Li:** When *qi* fluctuates it can both drain and boost your *shen.*

**Lu:** Then what does strong *shen* do *for* us and weak *shen* do *to* us?

**Zhong-Li:** When *shen* is strong your health is robust, your mind is resolute and life expectancy is long. But when *shen* is weak, so are you.

**Lu:** Is *shen* unique to each individual?

**Zhong-Li:** *Shen* is the same in everyone and every living thing. A whole army can have *shen,* and when this is the case, they become invincible. The great Chinese general Marshall Yueh Fei trained his army diligently with a martial form of *daoyin* called "Eight Strands of the Brocade" and never lost a battle.

**Lu:** So *shen* will help you achieve your goals in life?

**Zhong-Li:** It will do more than just that; it will sustain your mental and physical health, for without your health you have nothing.

**Lu:** What role does *shen* take on the longevity path?

**Zhong-Li:** Shen is the beacon that lights up the path and drives us onward. It is the source of motivation and inspiration, and the further you progress on your journey the stronger the *shen* becomes.

**Lu:** Which is more important: the refinement of me or *shen* to complete the Earth Path?

**Zhong-Li:** When an adept has evolved in a personal and spiritual way to complete the Earth Path, new paths open up. These are the Middle Path and the Celestial Greater Path, in that order. This is because only by the navigation of one does the next material-ize. Without consistently refining yourself, the path you are on will be your limit.

**Lu:** How then do I refine my *shen* and walk all the paths of enlightenment?

**Zhong-Li:** Remember the principle of *wuwei,* "to do by non-doing"? To even attempt to refine your *shen* sets you up for failure, because *shen* is untouchable and needs no refinement; you are simply its vessel. It is *you* who must elevate to discover *shen* and its immense potential.

**Lu:** So by effortlessly staying the course sequentially on each of the three paths, and concurrently refining *me* to become more attuned to Yin and Yang, my personal *shen* will shine its light a little brighter at the end of each stage of my journey.

**Zhong-Li:** Yes.

# Spirit Guide Reveal

*Approximately 20 years ago, during sleep, I was offered a vision for the future that involved, arguably, the most famous of the historic tai chi masters, Yang Chen Fu. He was standing (see Figure 7) in Horse Stance (Ma Bu) wearing a traditional tai chi suit that was to my surprise brown in colour. On his shoulders, forming a human column and also wearing brown suits, were maybe 10 associates. I was astounded by how powerful Master Yang's legs were to support such weight and equally, how solid, stable, and earthed he looked.*

The distinct impression I took from this vision was that if your posture is structurally correct and aligned with the forces of the Tao, almost superhuman strength can be experienced. The other thing was that I felt that they were trying to tell me to "connect to earth" in order to "connect to the heavens."

Some years later, when I had started training with Grandmaster Dr. Yang, Jwing-Ming, he made sense of the message my guides had implanted into my mind when he said, "Only through a strong root can the *shen* be strong."

It is through the *shen* that we commune with the heavens to keep us mentally strong and, ultimately, become enlightened. But it is not only your mental strength that relies on having a strong root; your physical body needs the same.

During my early days of training with Grandmaster Michael Tse, I asked him what the difference was between Western students and his native Chinese (Hong Kong).

He replied: "Westerners' legs are weak, and this makes their bodies weak. Also, Chinese walk everywhere and squat down. This keeps their leg *qi* strong, and they don't suffer with back conditions like Westerners do."

In the pursuit of "dying healthy," leg strength is vital, especially in later life.

Incidentally, a few weeks after I had this special dream, I discovered through my Chinese teachers that in olden times the standard colour of the Yang family's training attire was, in fact, brown, (I never knew this prior to the experience).

# Conclusion

Hopefully, from this step, you will come to realize that you have a hidden force within that is with you all your life and working tirelessly behind the scenes to keep you both mentally and physically strong. It is a force that can be suppressed by poor life choices, yet can fill you and protect you if positive healthy choices are made. You only have to become aware. Create the conditions, and *shen* will do the rest.

# Step 8

# Eight *Daoyin* Longevity Exercises

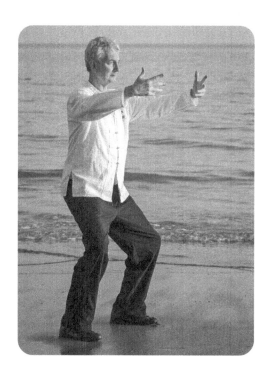

Here we are, at the final step of the Earth Path, where you physically reprogramme your body to help it help you. You are now at the threshold of the Middle Path, but only after spending the next few months practising what unfolds below.

As always, if you have an ongoing health issue you should discuss your intentions with your doctor before commencing the routines. You are also advised to contact your local qigong and tai chi associations, which will help you find a qualified instructor in your region. The human body is an amazing mechanism, capable of self-healing minor all the way to severe conditions, and the Eight Steps release its potential to the point:

> *When the mind, body, and spirit are free and uncluttered,*
> *Do nothing, for they know what to do.*
> ~ Taoist precept

"They know what to do"—to keep your body in a state of *homeostasis*, or perpetual lifetime balance: physically, mentally, and spiritually. The Tao is constantly working to maintain order and help you to live as long as your genes will allow, but for some unfathomable reason many people seem to be determined to interfere with this magical inner self-calibration.

Here is a reminder of the meaning and benefits of *daoyin*. It translates to mean "to induce (lead) and guide," which refers specifically to what the unique and meaningful exercises are able to do for the practitioner when mind and body are united.

Written references to *daoyin* date back some 2500 years, and in the late Han Dynasty (206 BC–AD 220) physician Hua Tuo prescribed *daoyin* for respiratory and digestive system ailments, arthritis and rheumatism, circulatory and heart conditions, and depression and general fatigue. Also in the Tang Dynasty (AD 618–907), physician Sun Si-Miao recommended it for all ailments, including infertility and impotency.

## Advice before Starting

- Do not attempt these exercises within one hour of eating a heavy meal.
- Wear loose-fitting clothing, and remove belts with heavy buckles.
- Practise in bare feet, if possible; otherwise, wear good quality trainers/sneakers.

- Do a few simple warm-up exercises, especially for knees and hips.
- The ideal location is outdoors in a warm and gentle climate with fresh air.
- Delay your practice if you are feeling fatigued.
- Take particular note of the advice given on posture in each exercise.
- Learn one exercise to a comfortable level before moving on to the next.
- Do not over-exercise; too much of anything can be bad for you. Keep to the advice given, and view this as physical medicine—just the right prescribed amount will heal.
- If you are new to this type of training, it is likely you may find it difficult to re-create the exact depth of shapes demonstrated in the illustrations. This is perfectly natural, and you should allow yourself time to assimilate the motions into your muscle memory. In time, you will naturally cascade down from "large circle" to "medium" then "small circles," as your body frame and muscles adapt.

### Daoyin 1

# The Hundred Arm Swings

*(Yibai Shoubi Baidong)*

There is an old saying in the UK, "An apple a day keeps the doctor away." In the same way that the apple is promoted for maintenance of health, the Hundred Arm Swings is prescribed to do the same.

Placed in the No. 1 position, this exercise is superb at loosening the body, generally, and is one of the ancient Heaven and Earth routines. It is perfect for preparing your body for any physical demands and, in ancient times, was prescribed to be repeated 100 times every day to ensure success in longevity.

In practice, you should start with 24 arm swings and over many weeks build up to 100 swings, spread throughout the day.

## Technical Performance

1  The first posture to perform in this exercise is Stand Still (1), which is designed to create the perfect launching position by aligning the feet with the shoulders (centre of the feet match centre of the shoulders). While in this posture, start by just swinging your pelvis (waist) forwards and backwards, without bending the knees. Let the arms naturally follow the swing of the pelvis; when both arms and pelvis are moving in unison, then you are ready to move on to posture 2.

2  Breathing in, swing the waist forward, and lift the chest, then the head, and swing the arms upward to the shape depicted in posture 2. The wrists should be raised to the height of your nose, with the elbows slightly tilted out and bent, not too straight.

3  From posture 2, commence breathing out, and sequentially lower the body; knees bend gradually in an outward curving motion, as this follows the natural tracking of the knee joints, which protects,

strengthens, and regulates the posture. In conjunction with this the chest lowers, shoulders lower, and head and elbows lower together. Fall gently under control and onward into posture 3.

4 Let the arms naturally swing down and back into posture 4. (Check the downward trajectory arm swing against supplementary imagery for the Hundred Arm Swings posture below: S1B, S1C, and side view in S1D.)

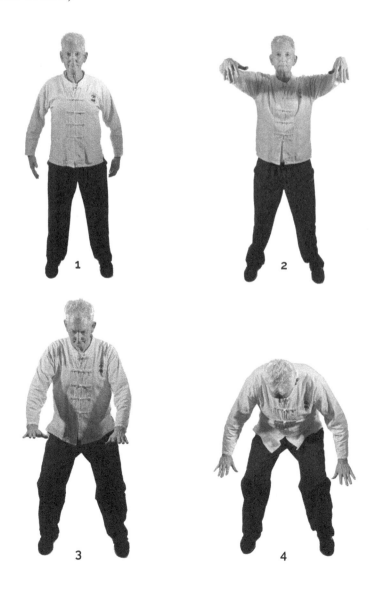

Step 8

# Sensory Performance

1 Stand for 30 seconds in posture 1, "breathe long" and visualize yourself standing on a mountain peak, feet firmly rooted to the solid mountain rock and your head lightly touching the heavens.

2 While in posture 1, bend the knees a little, and push from your feet as you breathe in, concentrating on the deep centreline running up the middle of the torso, neck, and head. Feel the subtle connection between your feet and your vertical core, and when you move on to perform the whole routine, retain this sense of the feet supported by the knees, influencing your upward and downward motions.

3 The resultant rising wave from the feet will raise your chest and head naturally, lifting the arms towards posture 2. If performed correctly, this should feel completely effortless, as if your whole body is floating up into the heavens.

4 As the arms rise, you should feel a sense of lightness, weightlessness, expansion, and fullness throughout the whole upper body. Upon reaching the summit of the upward arm swing as seen in posture 2 and S1A, you should slow everything down as your lungs reach full inflation. You are now experiencing being fully enveloped by the Heaven force of Yang.

5 While holding posture 2 just a couple of seconds, start to gradually bend your knees into Horse Stance, and breathe out slowly, as your body and arms (in that order) descend into position S1B. Sense the change within your body from light and expanded in posture 2 to gradually becoming heavy and deflated (but still retaining good structure) as you progress down into posture 3.

6 Keep breathing out as you continue to descend into posture 4, and feel the difference between how you felt in posture 2 (light, weightless, expanded, and full) compared to how you feel now as you enter posture 4 (heavy, rooted, semi-deflated, and empty). You are now experiencing your body being enveloped by the earth force of Yin.

7 As you flow between postures S1C and S1D (posture 4), create a natural bounce, which will help you rise almost effortlessly back up, and do not forget to use the breathing to support the motion all the way up and all the way down.

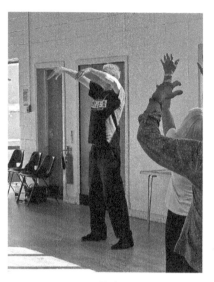

S1A

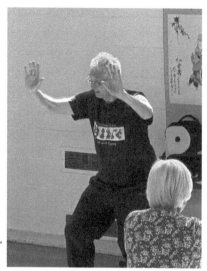

S1B

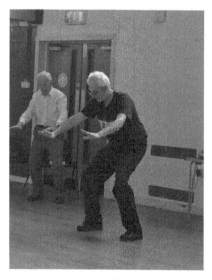

S1C

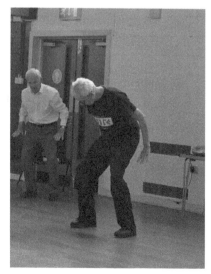

S1D

# Benefits for Health and Longevity

- There are two speeds (frequencies) to perform this routine: slow (to match long breathing) and moderate (not to match the breathing). The slow method will calm the whole system and generally regulate your circulation (fluid and electric). The moderate will invigorate the body, wake up the circulatory system, and offer a safe cardiovascular and respiratory workout.
- When the arms swing in conjunction with the spine extension and flexion, it releases tension throughout the whole upper body.
- It is a known fact that the ancient Chinese would swing their arms to get rid of headaches, because this would release muscular tension in the scalp, neck, upper back, upper chest, and shoulders (most headaches are caused by muscular tension).
- The range of movement in the natural arm swings clears stiffness in both shoulders.
- The combination of lowering the body to the earth and pushing upward to lift it to the heavens is particularly good for firing the piezoelectric in the structural bones. This, in turn, keeps the marrow healthy and strengthens the bones.
- The shape made at the top of the motion in position 2, opens the chest cavity, allowing the diaphragm to drop and the lungs to fully expand, creating healthy oxygen absorption (respiration).
- The shape made at the lowest point of the motion in position 4, helps the chest cavity to naturally close, assisting the diaphragm to spring back up and naturally deflate the lungs, creating healthy carbon dioxide expulsion (respiration).

# Note of Caution!

If you are undergoing treatment for lymphedema or any heart-related condition that impairs circulation to your limbs, you should only perform the slow version of the routine.

## Daoyin 2

# Beautiful Lady Rotates the Waist

### *(Piaoliang Xiaojie Xuanzhuan Yaobu)*

This routine comes from past and present China. Having to spend many hours of back-aching work in the rice fields, planting and harvesting rice crops, Chinese women would (and no doubt, still do) intermittently stop and perform this exercise to ease their backs. To this day the Chinese tai chi and qigong masters teach the exercise in the exact same way as it was performed thousands of years ago. Although its purpose is to release muscular tension and stiffness in the waist and lower back, it also offers benefits to hips and even ankle joints due to the rotational action of the waist over feet; the feet are to be shoulder-width apart and pointing forward.

## Technical Performance

1  From Stand Still posture, place the back of the hands on the lower back (or the palms, if this feels comfortable), and commence circling the waist as seen in postures 1–4 on the next page, in a clockwise motion (looking downwards).

2  The circles should be performed as 24 repetitions clockwise and 24 anti-clockwise, and each circle should match one respiration cycle. The breathing cycle should match the rotation of the waist, so that you breathe in as you circle round the front as postures 1–2 and breathe out as postures 3–4.

3  The head remains relatively central and does not circle around; the focus should clearly be only on the waist circling, which should form a perfect circle.

4  The knees should be held straight but relaxed, with some limited flexing to facilitate the circling of the waist and to help relax the hip joints.

**5** In this and all other *daoyin*, it is important to make sure that your feet are pointing straight ahead, shoulder-width apart, and perfectly parallel to each other. By doing this, you are ensuring that your knees, hips, pelvis, and spine are all correctly aligned for perfection of motion.

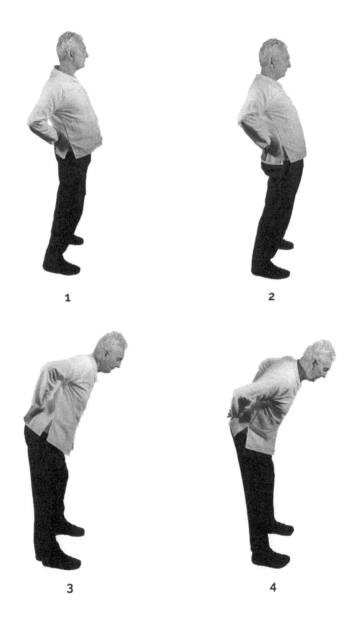

1

2

3

4

# Sensory Performance

1 In this case, I do not suggest that you visualize yourself standing in a rice field up to your knees in water. Instead, start slowly rotating the waist to create a perfect circle of clockwise motion (looking down at your waist to visualize the *tai chi tu* symbol), driven by the breathing.

2 As you circle to the front, let the breath fill the motion, as seen in S2A, B, and C (Yang) overleaf. As you circle to the back, let the breath empty from the motion as seen in S2D (Yin). Yang breathing supports the rising actions of the body, while Yin breathing supports the lowering actions.

3 The waist soft tissues should feel as if they are performing a Mexican Wave-type action, which releases muscular tension and creates muscular equilibrium.

4 The knees must be kept generally straight but also relaxed and slightly flexing. This will aid the natural rotation of the hips/waist, and in addition, you should feel the rotation of the waist down into the gliding ankle joints.

5 If sitting, you should firmly plant both feet on the ground and push upward from the feet to drive the upright circling round the back in posture 2 and breathe in (Yang). Then as you circle round to the front in posture 3, switch off the power from the feet, and just let your body almost fall into the front circling, and breathe out (Yin).

# Benefits for Health and Longevity

- Eases lower back pain centred on the lower lumbar and sacroiliac joints, which rely on regular exercise stimulation to remain free-flowing and functioning.
- Helps regulate the lower abdominal organs as it flows between opening and closing the abdominal wall muscles. As you circle to the front into Yang, the organs open and separate to allow fresh

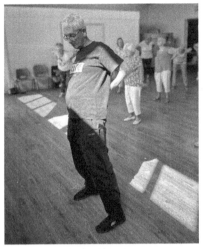

S2A

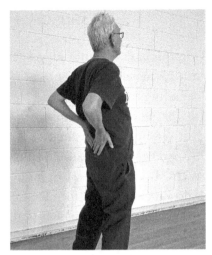

S2B

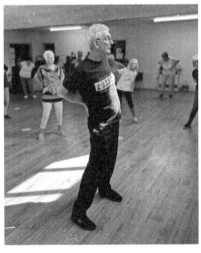

S2C

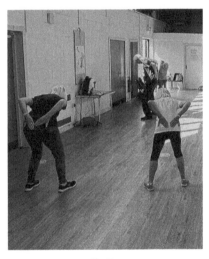

S2D

oxygen-enriched blood to flow through. And as you circle to the back into Yin, this contracts the organs back in creating a gentle, squeezing effect washing out any stagnant blood and toxins.

- Clears the girdle vessel (*dai mai*) meridian, which loops around the waist and is linked to the immune system, and it also supports all the other *qi* meridians of the body. The girdle vessel plays a major role in servicing the outer body shield known as the Guardian *Qi*, which is also believed to be associated with the immune system.

- If practised slowly and in harmony with breathing, it helps the diaphragm to move through its required full range of movement. This maintains the elastic properties of the diaphragm and slows its degeneration through aging.
- The ankles also benefit from the rotational waist movement, which indirectly regulates the gliding surfaces of the ankle joints.
- By circling the waist over the fixed feet, you are subtly improving your sense of balance, which is allowing you to move your upper body through a reasonable range of motion while remaining rooted to the ground.

**Daoyin 3**

# Three Powers
## *(San Tsai)*

*Daoyin 3, San Tsai* or Three Powers, is fundamental to successfully completing the Earth Path, because a human without the "three powers" is someone who is structurally, mechanically, mentally, and spiritually impotent. The "three powers" are Heaven, Earth, and YOU.

The goal with this *daoyin* is to make you the "third power" by falling gently and naturally to Earth (squatting), then extending the whole body upward and outward (maximum Yang) to Heaven. After this, the third power materializes when you fall naturally back to earth into Stand Still neutral posture, creating within your body a perfect balance between Heaven and Earth.

> *They must stand with their heads against the sky*
> *And have their feet rooted in the earth.*[49]
>
> ~ Zhong-Li

## Technical Performance

1 Starting in posture 1 (neutral), breathe in and lower yourself into *Ma Bu*—Horse Stance, and partially exhale, maintaining a straight spine, as shown in posture 2.

2 Continue to sink into posture 3, and release what is left of the breath.

3 Slowly and gradually push the body up to posture 4, breathing in as you rise. Then allow the body to fall naturally back into posture 1 as you breathe out. Initially, repeat the full routine four times, and build to a maximum of eight times.

4 Throughout this Heaven and Earth routine, it is important to remain as structurally aligned as possible as you move between each of the four postures.

5 When moving between each posture, you should stay calm within and as steady as possible, so that each transition shows no sign of weakness.

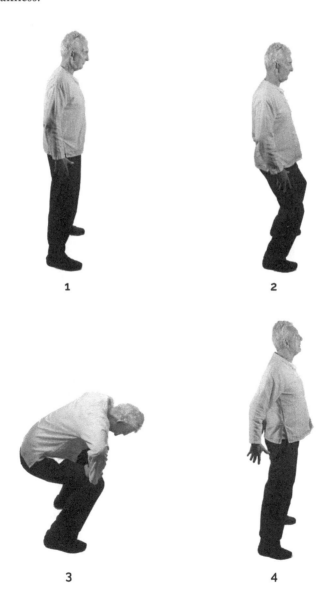

1

2

3

4

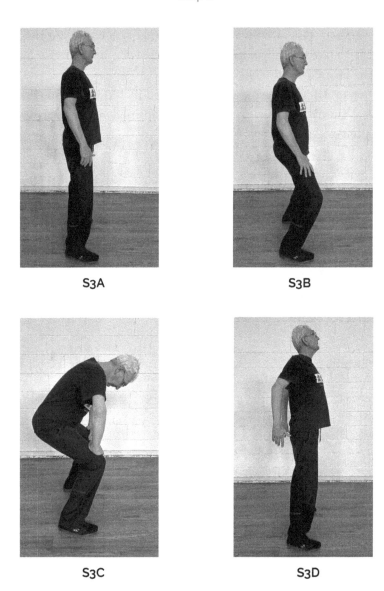

S3A                    S3B

S3C                    S3D

## Sensory Performance

1 This time, visualize yourself standing inside a transparent *tai chi tu* symbol (see opening image of Daoyin 3), conscious that the top half of your body (from the navel up) is light and gravitating upwards to correspond with Yang on the symbol. Now sense the lower half of

the body (from the navel down) is heavy and naturally gravitating to the earth, which is Yin on the symbol. With this in mind, stand for a while in posture 1 to gather your thoughts and calm your mind before commencing the routine.

2 Breathe in and out gently through the nose to regulate your breath for "long breathing."

3 Feel the out-breath assist the lowering of the body into postures S3B and C; lower the head to look down to the earth as you slide down into C.

4 As you land in posture 3/S3C, create a springy tendon bounce to help you rise to posture 4 while gradually breathing in. The head should slowly lift up to form a "Gazing at the Moon" shape which serves to open your airways and elevate your *qi*.

5 To finish, you should feel the out-breath lower you from posture 4 back to posture 1, which is regarded as returning to neutral and settling.

## Benefits for Health and Longevity

• This trains you to return to operating the natural mechanics of motion when bending and straightening up, also known in tai chi circles as "moving in folds."

• Retaining the deep gravity line through the centre of all movements has a stabilizing effect and prevents excessive localized loading of the body (too much weight focused in one area), which impacts the normal healthy functioning of organs, muscles, and joints.

• The bones are condensed and neutralized, which fires up the piezoelectric effect (electrical charge) in the structural bones (spine, pelvis, femur, tibia, fibula, ankles, and feet), thereby improving bone density.

• A sense of whole body balance appears which stays with you well into old age, lessening the risk of falls. This is so important due to the number of people who die prematurely as a result of falls.

- It is particularly good for regulating all the circulatory systems of the body, which rely on you retaining good posture, even when your body is in motion.

*Three factors (Powers) serve to complete*
*Heaven, Earth, and Man (Mankind).*[50]

~ Nei Ching

**Daoyin 4**

# Great Bear Spine-Stretching

*(Daxiong Shezhan ta de Jichui)*

This gem of a routine was inspired by the actions of a large bear that marks its territory in the wild by standing on hind legs with its back to a tree and stretching itself up as tall as it can, only to bite a chunk out of the tree bark. Any other bear that wanders into the first bear's territory will check out the rival by repeating what the first bear did, and if it finds the original tree bark bite is higher than it can reach, it vacates the region for fear of encountering the larger bear. Note! The author has seen everything described above in a TV documentary on wild bears.

It is also known in qigong as Spine Wave and Organ Massage, which describe the additional benefits this routine offers. The natural cyclic rise and fall of this routine concentrates the Yin and Yang vapours so that they flow in harmony throughout the body along their true pathways.

## Technical Performance

1 Start by performing a small shoulder girdle rotation in a forward direction, then coordinate it with the postures shown overleaf.

2 Breathe in as you rotate the shoulders upward, and breathe out as you rotate the shoulders down through postures 2 and 3.

3 From posture 3, roll the shoulders underneath to raise the back through posture 4, and slowly breathe in as you come up to posture 1 again. Continue the full cycle eight times.

4 The principle postures demonstrated in Daoyin 3 (Three Powers) are the core of this routine.

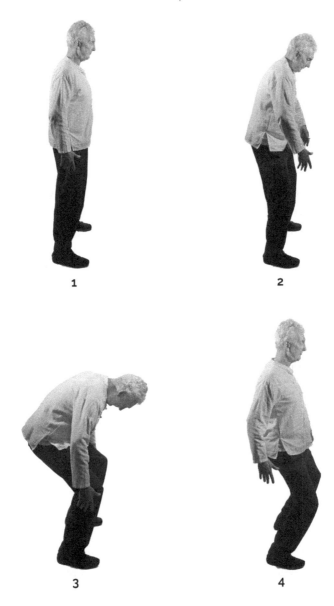

1                    2

3                    4

## Sensory Performance

**1** Visualize yourself as a rising ocean wave gaining momentum as it
rushes towards the sloping beach. The wave crests, crashes on the
beach and slides ever so subtly back into the ocean, from where

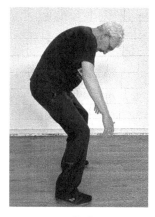

S4A

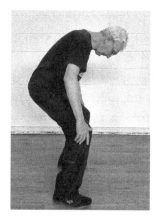

S4B

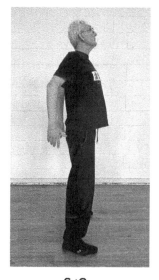

S4C

it gathers its strength to commence the cycle again. To start the process, practise the shoulder-rolling with the eyes lightly closed, and sensitively link the rising shoulder action with the in-breath and the descending action with the out-breath.

2 Now sense and feel how the small cog of the shoulder rotation marries to the big cog of the whole body in the Great Bear Spine-Stretching routine.

3 As you breathe in at the top of the routine (S4C), sense the expansion and lightness of Yang, while being aware of the spine now in full extension.

4 As you breathe out in the descending phase (S4A), sense and feel the emptying and deeply relaxing Yin appear and how it gradually returns to a rising spine-wave action in Yang between postures S4B and S4C.

# Benefits for Health and Longevity

- It develops a sense of coordination through the core of the body, from the soles of the feet to the top of the head.
- It encourages "long breathing," along with all its accompanying benefits (see Step 2) and is also known as Dragon breathing (Long *Huxi*), because a dragon breathes mechanically by rippling its spine.
- It moves the spine in a wavelike action that enhances circulation of the cerebrospinal fluid and synovial fluid, which are essential for a healthy spine and nervous system.
- If kept intimately linked to "long breathing," it will help regulate blood pressure. For example, to gently raise low blood pressure (hypotension), perform as shown; to gently lower high blood pressure (hypertension), simply reverse the whole process by rotating the shoulders backward and downward in an opposite circle to that illustrated. **Note:** Practising both methods is recommended, as it will encourage homeostasis of the body's circulatory systems.
- As noted, in some Taoist quarters, specifically to do with qigong, Great Bear Spine-Stretching is known as the Organ Massage exercise due to the rhythmic wave action of the spine/torso. This action compresses the organs as the body lowers into Yin, then releases and opens them to circulate fluids and *qi* life force as the body rises into Yang.

**Daoyin 5**

# Swaying Bear
## *(Yaobai Xiong)*

This exercise is designed to loosen and regulate the three zones of the body: lower torso, mid torso, upper torso, and head. Bears sway when they are threatened, and obviously it was this behaviour that was witnessed by the ancient Chinese more than 2300 years ago, when Chuang-tzu, in *The Book of Master Chuang* (circa 369–286 BC) wrote: "Swaying like a bear is only for longevity."[51]

## Technical Performance

1 Lower the body into posture 1, forming a shape reminiscent of hugging a tree (see Great Bear Spine-Stretching posture 2, page 152). Commence swinging/swaying the arms left and right, as shown in postures 2 and 3, to a count of eight: left being one and right being two.

2 Tilt the torso up while standing in Horse Stance, as shown in postures 4 and 5, still hugging a tree, and swaying left and right to a count of eight. The hands should be opposite the centre of the chest (*shan zhong* point).

3 Straighten the legs, but keep the knees relaxed and able to flex. Then lift the hands to opposite the forehead, as shown in postures 6 and 7 (page 157), and sway eight times left and right; after which you zig-zag slowly back down to posture 1 to end the routine.

4 As you bring up in your mind the image of a bear in natural repose, note the roundness in the arms and legs that release the structural frame to flow and circulate.

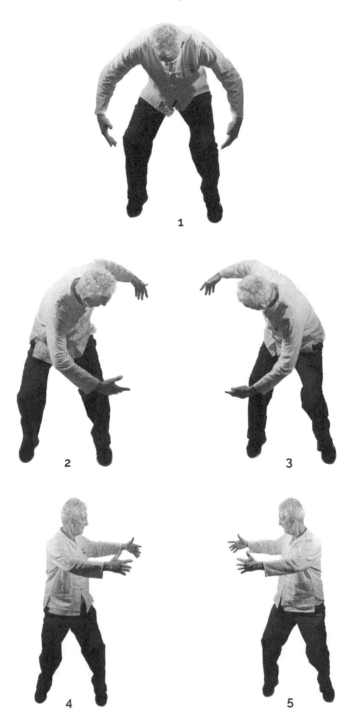

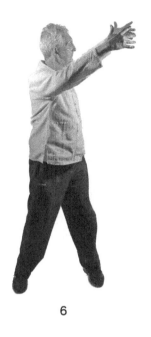

6

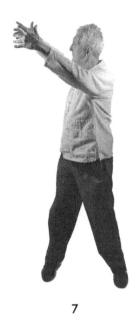

7

## Sensory Performance

1  In this routine, it helps to see yourself as a bear standing upright (go online and look for images), observe the relaxed, open, and rounded powerful posture of the bear. The swaying throughout the routine is best performed at a medium pace without the need to match the movements with specific breathing.

2  Develop a natural swing that is almost effortless to perform, while being conscious of your torso muscles remaining relaxed (see S5A and S5B overleaf for a guide).

3  Create a swaying motion in the arms by turning the waist as you push from the feet. This creates the integrated body motion necessary to elastically stimulate tendons and muscles from the spine outwards.

4  Sense and feel the muscles of the lower, middle, and upper back alternatively being stretched, especially where they connect to the spinal column. The greater the elasticity of the muscles and tendons, the more youthful you will remain.

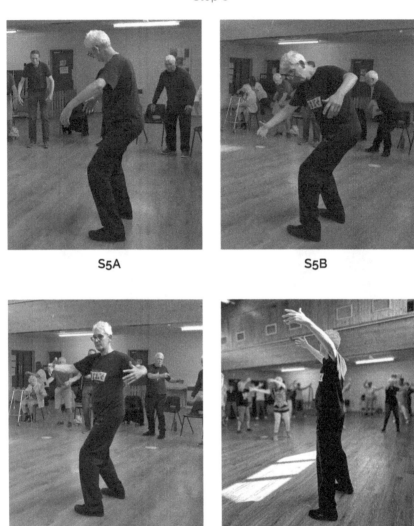

S5A

S5B

S5C

S5D

# Benefits for Health and Longevity

- Making the shape of hugging a tree opens the circulation in the whole body by rounding the limbs, thus removing the kinks in the circulatory systems.
- The swaying action through the three zones removes stiffness in the soft tissues of the core/torso generally.

- Swaying (horizontally turning) the spine along with flexion (bending) and extension (straightening) eases all the major joints and core structural muscle attachments of the sacrum and lumbar and thoracic vertebrae of the spine.
- It will help regulate blood pressure by relaxing all the soft tissues, which encourages free flow of the circulation, and by doing so, removes the pressure build-up in the system.

**Daoyin 6**

# Support the Heavens
## *(Tou Tien)*

Visualize the Support the Heavens exercise as similar to the Three Powers routine: you become one with Heaven and Earth, only this time with your hands holding up the sky. Support the Heavens is probably the most famous longevity exercise ever created, depicted for thousands of years in both Taoist and Buddhist longevity imagery. It has numerous health benefits, including mental health, and according to the ancient masters, should be practised daily in order to "live long and die healthy."

## Technical Performance

1  From posture 1, lower the body and make a scooping action that culminates with the shape seen in posture 2.
2  Imagine that you are lifting a bowl in front of the body. As your hands approach the upper chest, gradually rotate them 360 degrees, outwards with palms up, ending in posture 3. Hold the posture for a few seconds, then lower the arms to posture 4, flowing straight back into posture 2. Repeat eight times.

## Sensory Performance

1  In this *daoyin* exercise, you become the connecting conduit between Heaven and Earth, sensing how maximum Yang flows into maximum Yin, and vice versa. From posture 1, open the arms away from the body, and breathe in. Bend the knees, and breathe out, as you lower yourself into posture 2, and allow the body to feel as if it is emptying.

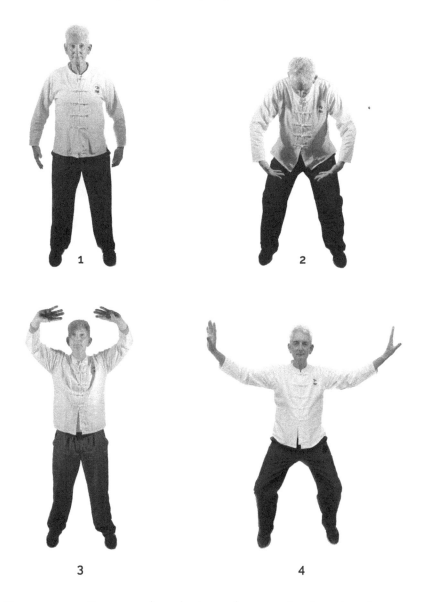

2  From posture 2, start to breathe in, and as you rise, imagine that
   you are drawing up earth *qi* through the whole body and out
   through the "sky eye," (see Figure 44 Yin Tang location, believed
   to be the psychic "third eye") as shown in posture S6A, pushing
   up the sky and forming a human conduit between Earth and
   Heaven.

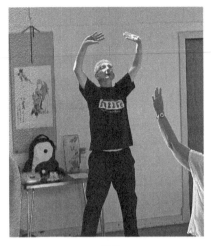

S6A

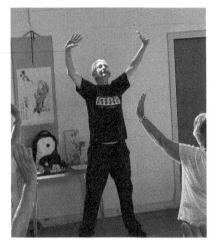

S6B

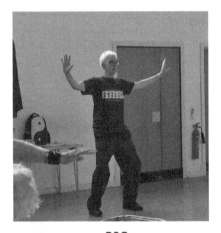

S6C

**3** Separate the hands slightly to form the posture shown in S6B, and feel as though you are now supporting the sky to prevent it from falling. In this position, hold the breath for a couple of seconds, then separate the hands even more into posture S6C, and commence breathing out until you arrive at posture 4.
**Note:** When separating the hands from posture S6A, imagine that you are parting the clouds and can see the mysteries of the universe.

# Benefits for Health and Longevity

- It tunes the whole body into universal *qi*, electromagnetic energy that is believed to create a healthy cellular body.
- It stretches the whole spinal column (maximum extension), then brings it to rest in recovery position (maximum flexion). This results in a healthy, balanced spine, with improved circulation of: synovial fluid, cerebrospinal fluid, and general blood supply.
- Because the arms are the "wings of the lungs," this exercise moves and coordinates the respiratory mechanics associated with the spine, ribcage, and diaphragm.
- This routine is a dynamic form of Three Powers training, and as such, you will develop a deep sense of postural balance between the forces of Heaven and Earth.
- After performing this routine (eight repetitions daily), you will feel a spirit of vitality throughout the body and a general sense of wellbeing. This is particularly good for your mental health.

## Daoyin 7

# White Crane Stretching
### *(Bai He Shenkai)*

All Chinese martial and healing arts have stretching as part of the curriculum, and longevity-based *daoyin* is no exception. The ancient Chinese observed nature in all its forms, and the red-crowned crane did not escape their attention with its graceful and natural contortions.

Over many centuries the Taoist observer identified a range of crane movements that could be linked to specific health benefits, including longevity. The White Crane Stretching Its Wings routine outlined here is made up of three parts. It would traditionally have been performed in the early morning when Yang *qi* is strong and fresh, and its other name is *shang wu* qigong, or morning exercises.

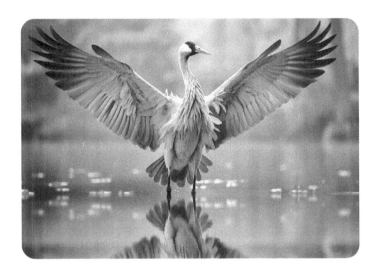

*Stretching like a bird [crane] is only for longevity.*[52]
~ Chuang-tzu

## Technical Performance—Three Parts

**Part One:** From posture 1, squat gently down into posture 2 (Sitting on the Earth), and push upwards from the feet to rise into posture 3 (Crane Stretches to the Heavens). Leave the arms and hands connected to the heavens, and start to bend the knees. This will create a pulling-down action on the arms, which should naturally lower into posture 4. **Note:** This exercise differs from the Hundred Arm Swings in that the arms just lift and do not swing up or down.

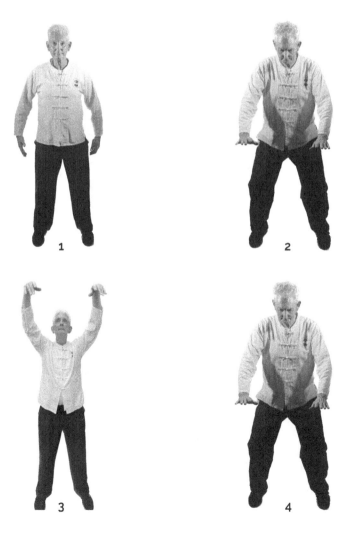

**Part Two:** Tilt your torso up while keeping the knees bent, and strike the pose shown in posture 5. Now, start to straighten the legs while extending the arms into posture 6 (Crane Stretches Its Wings Horizontally). Lean forward into posture 7 (Swooping Crane), keeping the legs straight, then bend the knees and return to Sitting on the Earth, as shown in posture 8.

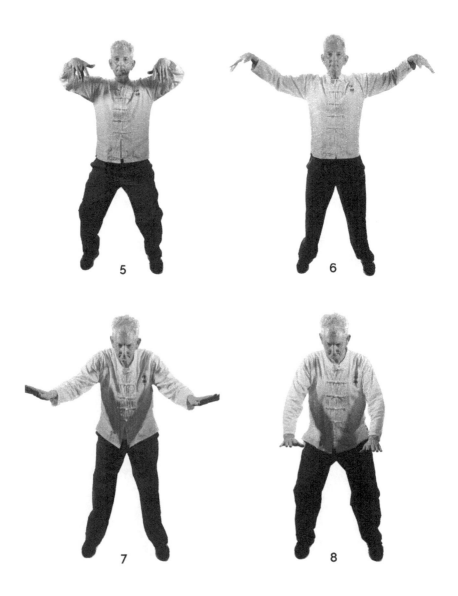

**Part Three:** From posture 8, leave your left hand facing down towards the earth, and tilt your body and right hand up to form posture 9. Now, slowly straighten your legs as you extend the arms into posture 10 (Crane Stretches Diagonally). Gradually bend the knees, and let the arms ("wings") fall naturally into posture 11. Now repeat the whole of diagonal stretching from posture 11 to posture 14, left side stretching upward (see postures 13 and 14 overleaf).

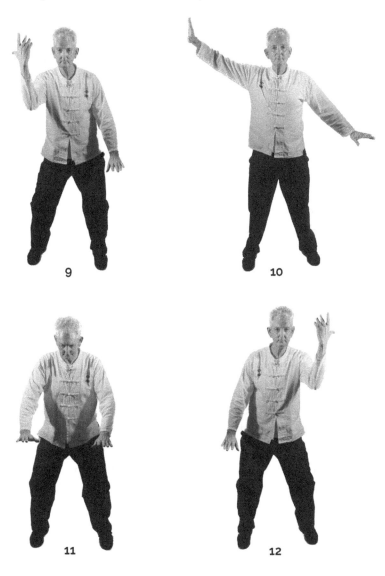

9

10

11

12

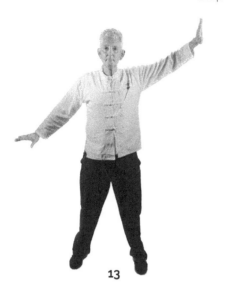

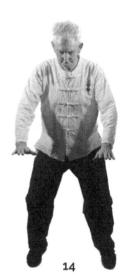

13

14

## Sensory Performance

In this exercise, you become a crane, imagining yourself moving with its grace and balance, allowing your senses to reach out to your wingtips (fingertips), while bowing your spine inward and outward, just as the crane does. Sense how your arms become the "wings of the lungs," and how they interact with the opening and closing of the lungs.

**Part One:** Breathing out, lower into posture S7B, and feel the empty force of Yin rooting you to the earth. Now, begin to breathe in as you push from the feet, and shunt the core of your body up to posture S7A, sensing the rising force of Yang sequentially lifting the pelvis, chest, and head (in that order), with the arms following. Focus the eyes above the distant horizon, while the back of your hands stretch up into the clouds. Bend the knees while still holding the breath and the upper body shape shown in posture S7A. Commence breathing out, and allow the pelvis, chest, head, then arms to fall and return to posture S7B.

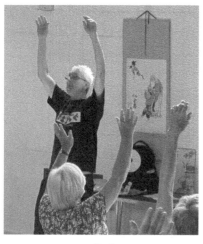

S7A

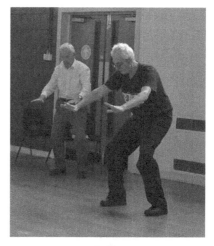

S7B

**Part Two:** Start breathing in, and continue through posture S7C to reach posture S7D. Feel as though your body and four limbs are filling with energized air (*qi*), and make an additional stretching movement to extend your arms out to your fingertips. Breathe out as you lean forward through posture 7, and arrive back at posture 8/S7B. For this last action, visualize that you are a crane swooping down to earth and landing.

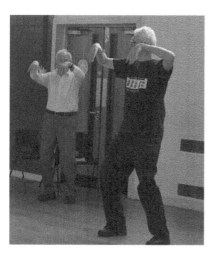

S7C

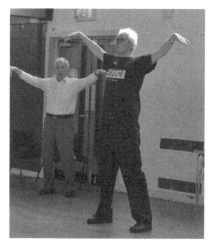

S7D

**Part Three:** From posture 8/S7B, keep the knees bent flowing into posture 9/S7E, and start to breathe in, continuing until you fully stretch out diagonally, as shown in posture 10/S7F. While holding posture 10, lift the chest and head a little higher, and inhale to top-up the lungs even more. Then bend the knees, and release the breath slowly as you lower the body and return to posture 11.

Perform the whole of Part Three again, but this time on the opposite side, as postures 12–14.

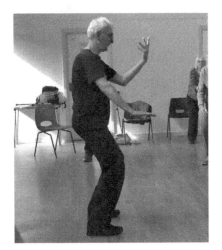

S7E

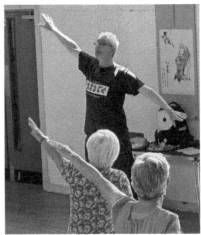

S7F

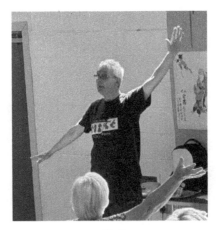

S7G

**Note:** When you stretch *(shenkai)*, you should not over-stretch, and when you relax *(huilai)*, you should not collapse. This creates equilibrium throughout the body, whether it is still or in motion.

## Benefits for Health and Longevity

**Part One:** This classic Heaven and Earth stretch opens up the whole body to breathe; that is, spine, organs, muscles, tendons, blood vessels, nerve fibres, and *jing lo*. It especially encourages the movement of oxygen-enriched blood to the brain, refreshing the cells, and fires up the piezoelectric effect in the structural bones through its condensing action.

**Part Two:** This is where Crane Airs Its Wings comes into play and where the expression "the arms are the wings of the lungs" makes sense. The perfect symmetry of arms ("wings") and body extending outwards while breathing in, floods the whole body with life-giving *qi*, awakening all the cells of the body. This is the best exercise for strengthening the whole respiratory system.

**Part Three:** This routine is designed for the expansion and contraction of alternate sides of the body, which means that, for example, if you have a weakness down the left side of your body you should perform more repetitions in that zone to strengthen it. As you extend outwards, focus your attention on the expanding side of the body (breathe into it), and it will energize. The mechanics of the arm movements are particularly good for the joints, lymphatic system, and general circulation throughout the limbs.

**Daoyin 8**

# Earthing Exercise
*(Jiedi Qigong)*

This ultimate *daoyin* exercise is placed here for good reason, because, according to the Great Masters, to progress further along the Earth Path you must "ground yourself and grow roots" to create the necessary stability of mind, body, and spirit *(shen)*. This final simple routine will provide the firm base on which you can build your longevity, because rooting is the foundation of a strong spirit *(shen)*, and without *shen* your journey will be fruitless.

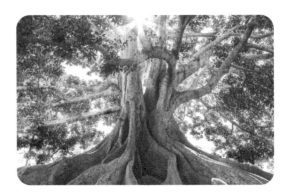

## Technical Performance

1 Stand in posture 1, and slowly lower the body into posture 2, leaning forward while looking down between your hands. The hands should press down and be parallel to the earth, elbows sunk and slightly bent.

2 Straighten back up to posture 1, and turn your waist, but not your feet 90 degrees to the left, as shown in posture 3. Bend the knees into Horse Stance, while pressing the hands down to the earth at the sides, as in posture 4.

3 Rise, and return to face front, in posture 1, then repeat the process described in instruction 1. Follow this by repeating the process in instruction 2, but instead, perform postures 5 and 6, turning 90 degrees to the right.

4 Return to posture 7, and finish in posture 8, after completing eight repetitions at each of the three locations.

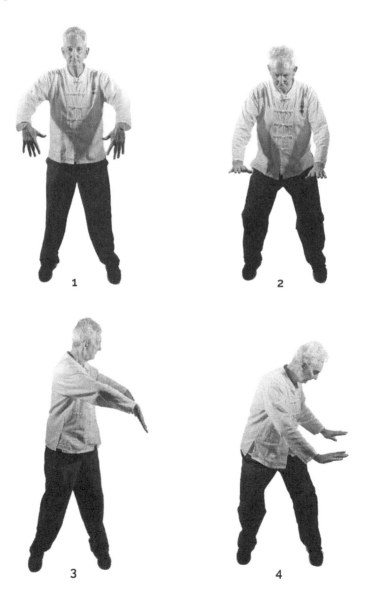

1  2

3  4

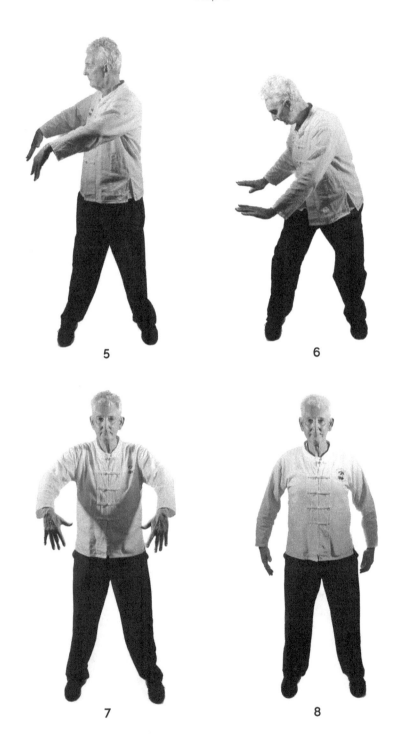

5

6

7

8

# Sensory Performance

There are two ways to sense rooting: The first is subtle, where you visualize yourself as a crane standing on a long bamboo shoot through which it is able to remain grounded by sensing its connect to earth along the bamboo stem; the second is when you imagine yourself as a strong, wizened, deeply rooted, old tree that has weathered many storms yet remains standing. Use the second approach as you perform this routine.

1  As you create the shape of posture 1/S8A, breathe in and sense your body and limbs filling and feeling light as they transform into Yang.

2  Bend your knees into Horse Stance, as shown in posture 2/S8B, and slowly breathe out as you sense your body and limbs emptying and feeling heavy as they transform into Yin. This is where you become the tree, with your roots planted deep in the earth, feeling especially heavy in your hands and feet.

3  As you rise from posture 2 and return to posture 1, breathe in and turn 90 degrees to your left into posture 3 while retaining the sense of fullness and lightness. Although the rooted heaviness you have just experienced lessens, some remains in the feet, while the whole upper body switches to Yang to become light and floating.

4  As you breathe out and lower your body into posture 4, press down to the earth while sensing your knees being gently pushed apart. This is known as "rooting to the side" and is an important technique for preventing falls.

5  Come back up on the in-breath, creating Yang, and slowly swing the upper body 90 degrees to start the process again, only this time turn to the right, as shown in posture 5/S8C.

6  Perform another "rooting" on the right side, as shown in posture 6/S8D, then go back to the beginning and repeat the whole routine seven more times, for eight in total.

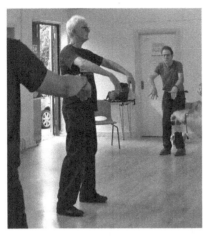

S8A

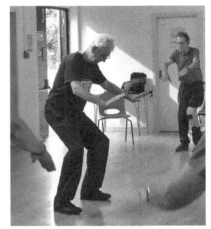

S8B

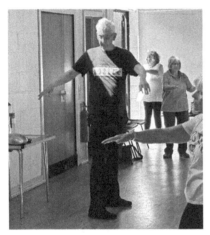

S8C

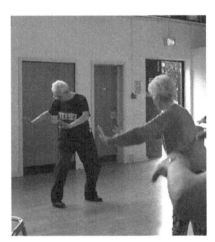

S8D

# Benefits for Health and Longevity

- It trains you how to develop the sense of breathing throughout the whole moving body.
- The sense of filling (*peng*) and emptying (*lu*) allows the general fluids (blood, lymph, synovial, and cerebrospinal fluids) and vapours (air and qi) to circulate freely and keep the body healthy.

- The fluctuation between expansion and contraction in the moving body creates a strong sense of "whole-body breathing" (*ti huxi*), allowing Yin and Yang energy transformation, which is essential for a healthy, long life.
- The central and peripheral nervous systems interact with one another, free from internal conflict. When the central nervous system has clear lines of interaction with the peripheral nervous system, it enhances proprioception (your body's ability to sense movement, action, and location, allowing communication with your surroundings).
- The "rooting" technique used in this routine promotes a clear connection between the brain and the earth through the body, maintaining structural stability and helping to prevent falls.
- The more the mind and body sense and feel connected to the earth, the stronger the *shen,* an essential driving force along the Earth Path.

## Zhong-Li and Lu Discuss *Daoyin*

**Lu:** Master, why must I practise *daoyin* every day? Isn't healthy diet, herbal infusions, and hill walking enough to allow me to progress to the Tao?

**Zhong-Li:** Walking, diet, and herbs have their place, but so too does *daoyin. Daoyin* rebuilds, restructures, and elevates the human body to reach higher levels of existence. They are part of the Yin and Yang rhythms of life, without which you cannot expect to develop a Rainbow Body.

**Lu:** What is a Rainbow Body?

**Zhong-Li:** Rainbows are perfectly symmetric and are born of the heavens and are rooted to the earth. Is it not said, where a rainbow touches the earth you will find treasure? In addition, rainbows are transparent and free from the opaqueness of negative *qi.* This is the desired condition in human form on the journey to enlightenment: a person who, through diligent practice, aligns with Heaven and Earth and cleanses the body of human weaknesses to the extent that they become transparent and lit with the radiance of *shen*.

**Lu:** Is *daoyin*, therefore, the key to attaining longevity?

**Zhong-Li:** *Daoyin,* when practised correctly, acts like a musical instrument tuner: It fine-tunes the mind, body, and spirit to the point where Yin and Yang flow unrestricted and raises it to new levels of existence. It is said that those who have reached this level have voices that ring as clear as a bell.

**Lu:** Master, I think you have just described yourself.

**Zhong-Li:** Yes.

# Conclusion

It is important to mention at this juncture that you are not meant to restrict yourself just to these eight gems of longevity. You should walk, swim, run, climb, play sports, and do anything else that keeps you active. However, with these exercises meshed into your daily life, you stand a greater chance of fulfilling the goal of health now for longevity later.

# Ask Sifu

# Q & A on Life and Longevity

The following questions are typical of those asked by newcomers and established students and are placed here to help you get the best result from this book.

## Total Integrated Body Motion

*Q: How and why do the Chinese tai chi masters move their bodies slowly in such a graceful way?*

**Sifu:** The Masters describe their beautiful, deeply coordinated motion as *chan su jin,* which translates to "silk-reeling energy." They talk of the joints and soft tissues being finely connected by a silk thread of *qi* that links the toes to the fingertips, and that when we move, it should be in a gentle and flowing manner so as not to snap the fine silk thread. In addition, when the joints mobilize, they follow a natural tracking motion along the deep, sculptured pathways of all joints that allow them to remain stable and healthy.

The Western engineered mind would describe this process as "total integrated body motion." When practised regularly, with a calm mind, multiple health benefits materialize. A typical example is described as follows:

*Silk-reeling tai chi integrates the whole body to create unrestricted circulation to the soft tissues.*

~ Tai chi medical

It is through this naturally attuned posture aligned with the forces of the Tao that the body arrives at the correct frequency. Visually, it is as if the performer is moving underwater, with the flow and grace of sea grass. It is totally captivating for those who witness it, and enlightening for those who experience it.

# Earth Path Completion

*Q: How will I know when I have completed the Earth Path?*

**Sifu:** On the internet, you will find an abundance of images and videos by tai chi and qigong experts performing their postures with grace, spirit, and mechanical correctness that you can use for a comparison. These are best viewed as a guideline not a replacement for training directly with a suitably qualified tai chi and qigong instructor. Even if the instructor does not teach the same exercise routines depicted in this book, you will still learn the fundamentals of posture, mechanics, breathing, and *qi* circulation. This will give you a foundation so that you can perform the Eight Daoyin exercises correctly.

After about 6–12 months, you will know whether you are making progress by how you feel mentally and physically compared with before.

# To Understand

*Q: Sifu, you often talk about how the ancients understood things. What does "understanding" mean in the ancient Chinese mind?*

**Sifu:** The ancients were intuitively attuned to nature, the human body, and their interactions in order to create an optimally functioning unit.

They understood the process needed to follow the road to longevity, and how to reach a point of understanding in their evolution, when the body, mind, and spirit unite, free from inner conflict, and operate in complete harmony, allowing enlightenment. After reaching this important milestone, they were then ready to guide others on the same path. This is what is meant by "understanding": when you know where you have gone wrong in life, and can see the same faults in others, who lack awareness of the impact of their unguided steps. Incidentally, Confucius is said to have reached the point of understanding at the age of 70. That is seven decades of learning, pondering, observing, and experiencing life before he became in an earthly sense "enlightened."

*The autonomous mind is imbued with understanding.*[53]

~ Lu Dongbin

## Too Much to Absorb

*Q: I have studied the Eight Steps in great detail and find that I am struggling to integrate everything you recommend into my life. What should I do?*

**Sifu:** Like all reference books, you should not read it like you would a novel. Instead, take from it what you can in small bites, step by step, and when you have digested the life-enhancing gems, take another bite, until such time as you have naturally and comfortably devoured the whole cake.

## Mysterious Universe

*Q: I notice in the book that you make a reference to the "mysteries of the universe." What does this mean?*

**Sifu:** If I knew what this means, it would no longer be a mystery. It has taken our scientists decades to plan, assemble, and position the

James Webb telescope, and only now are they beginning to discover what makes the universe tick. In this instance, however, seeing the mysteries happens not just with the eyes, for, according to Taoist and Buddhist practices, we are also able to see with our "sky eye," the Yin Tang point located in the centre of the forehead (also called the "third eye"). The Supporting the Heavens *daoyin* exercise is designed to open this psychic eye. Once it is open, you will be more intuitive and sensitive to the forces of nature (Tao) as they influence and permeate everything and everyone. The name the ancients gave these collective forces is "universal *qi*." Maybe, this is the "mystery" in the "mysteries of the universe."

## Learning by Fast Track

*Q: Can I accelerate my learning of the Earth Path so that I can start Middle Path training?*

**Sifu:** Everything you learn must be in keeping with the natural rhythms of the Tao; otherwise, you will only develop a facade with no heart. Your training should fall in line with the Yin and Yang life cycle (see Figure 44); under no circumstances, throw your Tao rhythm off balance. Everything in the universe has a particular frequency, and learning is no different. Find harmony within your life, and discover how your own frequency can alter as you absorb the new and cast off the old. Remember the old saying: "Patience is a Virtue."

## Uncomfortable Meditation

*Q: When I sit and meditate crossed-legged, it makes my back ache, which distracts me from the meditation. What do you think I am doing wrong?*

**Sifu:** To make a cross-legged, classic, seated *jing zuo* meditation pose more comfortable, place a semi-rigid, raised support under your bottom.

This will lift your pelvis and ensure that your hips are slightly higher than your knees. Structurally, this helps keep your spine straight and will eliminate the risk of developing back pain. Remember, when sitting you must pay attention to your sitting bones and centre your torso and head directly above them. I also suggest you try simply sitting on a straight-backed chair, as seen in Figure 12, and try not to run before you can walk.

*Those who rush to reach their goals*
*Will meet themselves on the way back.*

~ Sifu

## Blocked Midriff

*Q: When I breathe, even through the nose, I feel tightness in my midriff, as if I have hit a wall. Why is this stopping me from taking a long and deep breath?*

**Sifu:** The diaphragm is responsible for two-thirds of your breathing and is a sheet of muscle that separates the chest cavity from the abdominal cavity. There are many potential reasons why you are experiencing this:

- Muscular tension caused by physical overexertion affecting your core muscles.
- Your mind is stressed and distracted and not body-centred, which causes the diaphragm to tighten.
- Your posture is not body-centred, which creates an imbalance in your breathing mechanics.
- Your breathing is too forced, which will tighten the respiratory muscles.

A clear, calm, and stress-free mind (Yi) is reliant upon a structurally aligned, calm, and stress-free body; they are inseparable: one does not function efficiently without the other.

# Mobility Issues

*Q: I have limited mobility and a number of health problems and am unable to attempt the* daoyin *exercises shown in Step 8. How can I gain at least some of the health benefits you illustrate in the book?*

**Sifu:** You should focus on what you can do, instead of what you cannot. Remember, Zhong-Li says that it is all about attuning your life, your mind, and your body to the rhythms of Yin and Yang (the Tao). You should start your programme of self-enhancement by developing a subtle blend of sitting training (Yin) with some standing (Yang), if possible. If you cannot stand, just adapt what you can for sitting. Practice *jing zuo* daily, and move slowly (as if moving under water) at all times, encouraging long natural nose breathing to support your physical actions.

# Aching Joints

*Q: My joints ache every day, and I have recently been told that I have osteoarthritis. Would living my life according to the Earth Path help me?*

**Sifu:** The probable causes of osteoarthritis are stress, poor posture, poor body mechanics, and—something I would focus on—poor diet, especially in the form of excess refined sugar consumption, which may serve as a temporary energy boost but can create a lot of unpleasant side effects. Excess refined sugar intake:

- Raises inflammatory chemical levels in the blood, which damage organs and inflame joints.
- Is linked to type 2 diabetes. By cutting out sugar, you can make the body less insulin resistant.
- Leads to craving, overeating, and weight gain due to the addictive nature of sugar.
- Increases the risk of heart attack and stroke (heart disease).

- Can lead to unnatural increases in liver fat deposits (fatty liver disease).
- Promotes high blood pressure (hypertension).

It is also interesting to note that the Alzheimer's Society in the UK has recently reported that eating excessive amounts of sugar increases the risk of developing Alzheimer's Disease. On a personal note, I was warned away from consuming excessive sugar by my Spirit sifu approximately 30 years ago.

By following the daoyin exercises shown in Step 8, and the advice given beforehand, you will retain (or regain) a healthy metabolism well into later life, and also increase the levels of the body's own natural anti-inflammatory chemicals in your blood, which can help ease joint pain.

## Painful Knees

**Q:** *When I bend down to perform the squatting postures in the book, I find my knees complain. How can I stop this occurring?*

**Sifu:** The knees are the accelerators and de-accelerators of all the body's physical actions and are the switches that turn the body into Yang when straightening or Yin when bending. If your knees are misaligned, they are the most likely body part to wear out, especially when you consider the immense pressures that impact the knee joints. Always keep the knees structurally aligned with the feet, and perform the routines and postures accurately. Move slowly, especially when bending, and do not attempt the full squatting posture depicted. Lower your body with the out-breath, to help the gradually bending knees follow their natural tracking, and come back up with the in-breath, doing the same.

Incidentally, you should bend and straighten the knees through their full range of motion regularly (daily) while sitting to keep them lubricated and healthy.

# Back Pain and Constipation

*Q: I suffer regular lower-back pain and constipation. Painkillers and laxatives fail to get to the root of the problem. What do you recommend?*

**Sifu:** There are many reasons why you could be experiencing these conditions:

- The first and most obvious one is diet: Unhealthy, stodgy, convenience foods are known to cause stagnation in the normal, healthy functioning of the bowel.
- Another culprit is posture. When sitting, your head should lift from the crown and as a counter-balance your torso should be centred and earthed over your sitting bones, located at the underside of your pelvis. This allows the whole abdominal cavity to breathe and the rhythms of the Tao to regain control.
- When standing, to release the abdomen, according to Traditional Chinese Medicine, the Crown point atop the head must link to its opposite number, the Kidney 1 (*Yong Chuan*—Bubbling Wells) points located at the centre of both balls of the feet. This creates the same favourable conditions throughout the whole body as described above for sitting.
- The practice of walking with a body attuned to the Tao is particularly beneficial for the relief of lower-back pain and constipation, providing you do so in the following way:

  - Keep your head up.
  - Keep eyes focused on the distant horizon.
  - Open your armpits.
  - Swing your arms from the shoulders.
  - Stride moderately.
  - Step lightly.
  - Place heels gently but firmly.

- Walking for a minimum of 30 minutes after eating helps the whole digestive system to function, eases back pain, and regulates the bowels.

- A general rule for abdominal health is to keep your floating ribs high above the iliac crests (top) of the pelvis, whether you are sitting, standing, or walking. You will notice this keeps the lower abdominal space open so that it can regulate itself.
- In addition to all the above, you should naturally "long-breathe" into the abdomen (abdominal breathing), which is known to break down the solids in the bowels.

**Note:** If you are experiencing these specific symptoms, it is wise to first visit your doctor to eliminate any medical issues.

# Reoccurring Cystitis/ Urinary Tract Infections (UTI)

*Q: As a man, I thought that cystitis and urinary tract infections (UTIs) manifested only in females until I experienced one myself. After repeated visits to my doctor and countless antibiotics, I am still having regular flare-ups. Can you help?*

**Sifu:** Because of the way our male genital anatomy differs from females we are less likely to suffer from UTIs and cystitis; however, it still happens, and when a man looks into what is available in the form of treatment and advice, 99 percent is geared to women. Men seem to have been forgotten, despite many men suffering in silence. Here is a list of possible remedial options that may be of use to both men and women sufferers:

- Wear loose-fitting underwear, trouser/skirt waistbands, and belts. Anything that cuts into the bladder area will irritate the condition.
- Start an immediate low/no sugar diet, cutting out all sweets, chocolate, cookies/biscuits, cakes, ice cream, high sugar food, such as cereals and sugary drinks. Consuming natural unprocessed sugars at a low level is better, if needed.

- Stop all alcoholic beverages until symptoms have cleared.
- Avoid citrus fruits and drinks.
- Avoid coffee, hot chocolate, and tomato juice. Instead try rooibos (redbush) tea, chicory coffee, sugar-free dandelion coffee, and pure carob powder.
- Increase your intake of still mineral or tap water. Avoid sparkling water, which can irritate the system.
- Go to the toilet to urinate the moment you get the signal. Do not put it off as this can encourage the bad bacteria to multiply.
- Keep checking the colour of your urine. If it has gone cloudy and darkened to orangey-red in colour, drink a pint of water straight away and keep flushing until your urine has returned to a natural straw colour.
- Always maintain good posture in accordance with the advice in this book.
- If you have developed (and returned to) natural "long abdominal breathing," you can focus your breathing as if you are breathing through the whole bladder/UTI region. This massages the inflamed soft tissues so that they heal more quickly.
- The qigong and daoyin exercises described in this book will cleanse and calm the irritation. One of the main reasons for this is that exercise releases natural anti-inflammatory chemicals into the bloodstream.
- Avoid sexual activity until the symptoms have cleared, and even then, your activity should be moderate, never excessive. Remember to always urinate after sexual intercourse, and drink a pint of water to wash out the system.

**Big note:** All the above advice is given freely on the understanding that you check with your doctor about any persistent urinary conditions. If left unchecked, they could lead to a more serious kidney infection.

# The Die Healthy Experience

*Q: When, and if, I reach a ripe old age, how am I going to be functioning during the Die Healthy phase? I have no wish to be there if I end up relying on someone else to dress me, feed me, and so on.*

**Sifu:** The whole point of belabouring the maxim "Invest now for later life" is so that you can remain physically and mentally independent throughout your whole life. Based on the evidence provided in this book, you should by now understand that it *is* possible to be happy, contented, physically active, and relevant into your nineties, and in some cases beyond. I refer you to the following joint venture research findings by scientists at two universities in the Netherlands:

> *The maximum ceiling for a female lifespan is 115.7 years, and for men 114.1 years. This isn't about life expectancy but lifespan, which is used to determine how long a single individual can live as long as they look after themselves.*[54]
>
> ~ Tilburg University, Netherlands

Bear in mind that the above figures are based on individuals who take care of themselves through diet, exercise, and lifestyle, supported by improvements in medical science, and without the addition of the Earth Path training offered in this book. However, with this advice it will make the realistic journey so much easier, and you *can* expect a more favourable and independent outcome towards the end of your golden years.

# Final Comment of Ancestor Lu Dongbin

*Q: How do you know if you have completed the Earth Path?*

**A:** When illnesses gradually disappear and the body is light and comfortable, and when weaknesses and defects are repaired and one is physically and mentally strong and healthy.[55]

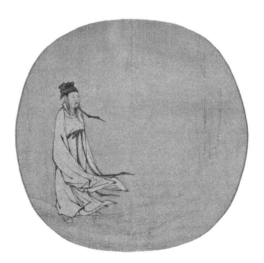

**Fig. 49** Ancestor Lu Dongbin
crossing Lake Dongting

# Notes

1   Dr. Charles Windridge, *Tong Sing: The Chinese Book of Wisdom* (London: Kyle Cathie Ltd, 1999), 50.

2   D.W. Winnicott, *Playing and Reality* (London: Routledge, 1991), 99.

3   Ted J. Kaptchuk, *Chinese Medicine* (London: Rider, 2000), 3.

4   Master B.P. Chan, in Kenneth S. Cohen, *The Way of Qigong* (New York: Ballantine, 1997), 134.

5   John Blofeld, *Taoism: The Quest for Immortality* (London: Unwin, 1986), 21.

6   Thomas Cleary, *The Essential Tao* (Harper San Francisco, 1991), 124.

7   *Journal of Neuroimaging,* official journal of the American Society of Neuroimaging (Hoboken, NJ: Wiley, 2018). National Library of Medicine. www.pubmed.ncbi.nlm.nih.gov/29667260

8   *AHA,* Journal of the American Heart Association (Dallas, TX: 2017). www.ahajournals.org/doi/10.1161/JAHA.117.006603#:~:text= Compared%20with%20a%20shorter%20intervention,declined%20 enrollment%20in%20cardiac%20rehabilitation

9   *Heart and Lung: The Journal of Cardiopulmonary and Acute Care* (Philadelphia, PA: Elsevier: 2020), www.doi.org/10.1016/j.hrtlng. 2020.02.041

10  Department of Nursing, (South Korea: Makpo Catholic University, 2009), www.doi.org/10.1080/00207450390245306, 1691-170.

11  Department of Clinical Psychology (Sweden: Uppsala University, 2009), www.doi.org/10.1080/09638280701400540, 625-633.

12  Kinesiology Department (Chicago, IL: University of Illinois, 2007), www.news.illinois.edu/view/6367/206578

13  *Annals of Oncology,* European Society of Oncologists (Amsterdam, Holland: Elsevier, 2009), www.doi.org/10.1093/annonc/mdp479, 608-614.

14  "Tai chi can help older patients with disabling conditions." (London: *The Guardian,* 2015), www.theguardian.com/society/2015/sep/17/ tai-chi-help-older-patients-disabling-conditions-study

15  National Library of Medicine (USA: PubMed, 2020), www.pubmed.ncbi.nlm. nih.gov/32839351/

16 *Harvard Health* (Cambridge, MA: 2013), www.health.harvard.edu/blog/
tai-chi-improves-balance-and-motor-control-in-parkinsons-
disease-201305036150

17 American Heart Association (Dallas, TX: 2013), www.heart.org/en/
healthy-living/fitness/walking

18 Dr. Yang Jwing-Ming, *Qigong Meditation.* (Boston, YMAA Publication Center,
Inc, 2003), 248.

19 Ilza Veith, *The Yellow Emperor's Classic of Internal Medicine* (Malaysia: Pelanduk
Publications, 1992), 97, 98, 101, 103.

20 Ibid.

21 Ibid.

22 Thomas Cleary, *The Essential Tao,* 9, 17.

23 D. C. Lau, *Lao Tzu Tao Te Ching* (London: Penguin Books, 1963), Book One,
p. 13, IX. 23.

24 Ibid. Book One, p. 34, XXIX. 68.

25 Ibid. Book One, p. 35, XXX. 70.

26 Ibid. Book One, p. 38, XXXIII. 75.

27 Ibid. Book One, p. 38, XXXIII. 75.

28 Ibid. Book Two, p. 53, XLVI. 105.

29 Ibid. Book Two, p. 61, LIV. 122.

30 Ibid. Book Two, p. 62, LV. 126.

31 Ibid. Book One, p. 31, XXVI. 59.

32 Ibid. Book Two, p. 65, LVIII. 136.

33 Thomas Cleary, *Vitality, Energy, Spirit,* 208.

34 Peter Newton, *Tai Chi & Qigong: The Ultimate Beginner's Guide* (Conwy, Wales:
China Bridge Publications, 2000), Classic 9: "Classics of Chang." 77.
www.chinabridgetaichi.com

35 Thomas Cleary, *Vitality, Energy, Spirit,* 212.

36 Peter Newton, *Tai Chi & Qigong,* Classics 6 and 10, respectively, 75, 78.

37 Ibid.

38 "Tortoise-Pigeon-Dog" (New York: *Time* magazine: May 15, 1933).
www.en.wikipedia.org/wiki/Li_Ching-Yuen

39 "The Chinese village with the secret to long life," (London: *The Guardian,*
30 December 2013). www.theguardian.com/world/2013/dec/30/
chinese-village-secret-long-life-bama-guangxi

40 James Legge, *The I Ching* (New York: Dover Publications, 1963), Appendix III, Section 1, Chapter 1, item 8, 349.

41 Eva Wong, *The Tao of Health, Longevity, and Immortality* (Boston: Shambhala Publications, 2000), 143.

42 D.C. Lau, *Lao Tzu Tao Te Ching*, Book Two, 49.

43 Yang Jwing-Ming, *Qigong Meditation*, 10.

44 Jou Tsung Hwa, *The Tao of Meditation* (New York: Tai Chi Foundation, 1983), 2, 3, 97, 159.

45 Norwegian University of Science and Technology (NTNU) "Brain waves and meditation." (Rockville, MD: ScienceDaily, 31 March 2010). www.sciencedaily.com/releases/2010/03/10031921631.htm

46 Thomas Cleary, *The Essential Tao*, 126.

47 Thomas Cleary, *Vitality, Energy, Spirit*, (Boston: Shambhala Publications, 1991), 74.

48 Ilza Veith, *The Yellow Emperor's Classic of Internal Medicine*, Book 1, 97.

49 Eva Wong, *The Tao of Health, Longevity, and Immortality*, 24.

50 Ilza Veith, *The Yellow Emperor's Classic of Internal Medicine*, Book 3, 135.

51 Thomas Cleary, *Vitality, Energy, Spirit*, xviii.

52 Ibid.

53 Thomas Cleary, *Vitality, Energy, Spirit*, 77.

54 "The oldest human does not get any older" (Netherlands: Tilburg and Erasmus universities, 2017), www.tilburguniversity.edu/current/press-release-/press-release-oldest-human

55 Thomas Cleary, *Vitality, Energy, Spirit*, 144.

# Glossary

*An:* "To press/push." In the context of tai chi chuan, it is when you apply a pushing action that gradually presses into the person's body through both hands using *qi* (subtle life-force energy) or *jing* (coarse physical energy) depending on whether it is for health or martial reasons.

**Ancestor Lu:** Lu Dongbin, also known as Lu Tung-pin, one of the famous Chinese Eight Immortals and reputed creator of the Earth Path.

*An Mo:* "Massage." This describes the technique of massaging the body by the actions of pressing, pushing, and rubbing.

*An Mo Qigong:* "Massage + Exercise." The practice of massage while performing gentle qigong exercise.

*Ba Duan Jin:* "Eight Strands of the Brocade." A powerful set of qigong exercises that have been attributed to two famous ancient Chinese Figures: Marshal Yeuh Fei, a Song dynasty (AD 960–1279) heroic general, and Zhong-Li Quan, one of the main subjects of this book.

*Bai He:* "White Crane." This refers to the majestic red-crowned crane, which features heavily in the arts of tai chi chuan and qigong.

*Bai He Huxi:* "White Crane Breathing." Believed to have been developed by the Shaolin monks of southern China, it involves combining movement of the arms with the spine to strengthen the breathing function.

*Bai Hui:* "One Hundred Convergences." The uppermost energy point (cavity) in the body; spiritually known as Heaven's Gateway.

*Chang:* "Long." Also known as *zhang*, an important principle in progressing through the Eight Steps along the Earth Path.

**Cheng Man-Ching:** Tai Chi Master Cheng Man-Ching gained fame in the United States during the 1960s for introducing tai chi chuan to the Western Hemisphere.

*Chi:* See "*Qi*."

**Confucius:** "Master Kong." The philosophical giant (551–479 BC) who, to this day, influences Chinese society and, to a lesser degree, is renowned worldwide.

**Confucian Analects:** A literary collection of the wisdom and sayings of Confucius thought to have been written by his disciples soon after his death in 479 BC.

***Dai Mai:*** "Girdle Vessel." Also known as the "Belt Channel," which is located in a loop around the waist. A strong Yang-balancing energy circuit that is linked to the immune system and helps keep the vertical meridians in harmony.

***Dan Tien:*** "Elixir field of energy." Located in three forward-pointing places on the body:

1 Centre of the forehead ("Sky Eye").
2 Centre of the sternum ("Middle Mountain").
3 Centrally one inch below the navel ("Sea of Energy").

They are collectively regarded as the three most influential and powerful energy points on the body.

***Dao:*** "The Way." It is often called "The Tao," which refers to the omnipresent original force of the universe that influences everything that exists, past and present. It is the root source of tai chi and the grandparent of Yin and Yang.

***Dao Shih:*** "Taoist priest." Originally believed to have evolved from the Fang Shih, the forbears of Taoist priesthood, they are still practising their ancient rituals to this day.

***Di:*** "Earth." Used in the context of Heaven and Earth.

***Du:*** "Spine-located Yang meridian, also known as the Governor meridian."

***Fajing:*** "Explosive power." Seen when the slow and graceful movements of tai chi chuan are speeded up and applied as a martial art.

***Fang:*** "To let go." Often used in the context of letting go of one's frustrations or inhibitions.

***Fangsung:*** "Relax and let go." It is the method used in tai chi and qigong to help empty the mind and body of tension and is the precursor to experiencing settling.

***Feng:*** "Wind." Found in the name of Chang San Feng, and used to describe acupuncture points high up on the back of the neck that are known to be susceptible to cold winds.

***Feng Shui:*** "Wind and Water." A broader form of geomancy practised by feng shui masters.

*Gong:* "To train." A term that can be attached to any discipline that requires dedicated practice.

**Hua Tuo:** A pioneer in surgery of the Han Dynasty (206 BC–AD 220) and regarded as the greatest surgeon in Chinese history.

*Huan Ying Hui Jia:* "Welcome home." Used in tai chi to describe when the body comes to rest in natural repose, creating a sense of returning home.

*Jiedi:* "Earthing." Describes the condition sought after in tai chi and *daoyin*/qigong.

*Jijing:* "Stillness." A condition much sought by Taoist adepts in cultivating the mind, body, and spirit.

*Jing:* "Course *qi*." Prenatal *qi* from your parents that is still present when you are born. Also one of the Three Treasures of Nei Gong: *qi, jing, and shen.*

*Jinglo:* "Energy body." A name to describe the meridian system of the body in acupuncture, part of Traditional Chinese Medicine.

*Kong:* "Empty." A term that refers to the meditative and physical state of mind and body respectively needed to explore the higher realms of the Taoist arts.

*Kung Fu:* "Chinese martial arts." Although it is widely known as a way to describe Chinese martial arts, it can also be used in the context of anything that requires a lot of: time, patience, and effort.

*Leng Ning Huxi:* "Condensing breathing." This is concentrated breathing that can be applied to specific organs, muscles, bones, and energy centres.

*Li:* "Physical Strength." Generally refers to the muscular power dynamics of the body.

*Lohan:* "Advanced adept." Someone who is on the cusp of attaining enlightenment.

*Long:* "Dragon." In China, the dragon is Lord of the Heavens and so revered that emperors were assumed to be their earthly manifestation. In addition there are five elemental dragons.

*Long Huxi:* "Dragon breathing." A wave-action type of breathing that circulates through the spine and enhances the whole respiratory system.

*Lu:* "Rolling back the *qi* to Earth." This comes from the application of tai chi chuan in self-defence and implies that you are guiding *qi* (subtle) and *jing* (physical) visible power to Earth, and is therefore associated with an outward-flowing breath.

*Mabu:* "Horse Stance." A posture where the feet are shoulder-width apart and the knees are bent, creating an upright, squatting posture likened to sitting on a horse. Used in Chinese martial arts and qigong/ *daoyin* as part of their therapeutic exercises.

*Mai:* "Vessels." Often seen written as *mei*, there are eight of these vessels in the body that store and regulate *qi*. They interact with the 12 main *qi* meridians.

**Mawangdui:** "King Ma's Mound." The burial place of Chancellor Li Cang, his wife Lady Dai, and their son during the Han Dynasty. It was from this tomb that the famous silk-screened *daoyin tu* images of Han people practising daoyin were found.

*Nei Dan:* "Inner elixir." This describes the *qi* that is channelled through the *Zheng Dan Tien* ("Real Energy Field") to create a powerful energy body.

*Nei Gong:* "Inner Gazing Training." Used in the internal development of healthy *qi* circulation.

*Peng:* "Ward off." Used in tai chi chuan to describe how *qi* (subtle) and *jing* (physical) power fills the body and creates a sense of outward expansion, served by an inward breath.

*Qi:* "Universal life-force energy." According to Taoist belief, *qi* is present in all living things. The ancient Chinese devised many methods to cultivate and enhance its presence in the body.

*Qigong:* "Energy training." An energy-based exercise system that is thought to have originated 5000 –7000 years ago in ancient China; also originally believed to have been called *Daoyin*.

*Qu Huxi:* "Zone breathing." A technique used to clear stagnation in areas of the body that would otherwise prove difficult to release.

*Ren:* "Human."

*Ren Mai:* "Human Conception Vessel." One of the eight Extraordinary Vessels that run down the front of the body and linked to the body's Yin meridians.

*Ren Ti:* "Human Body."

***Shiying:*** "To settle down." This is the sensitive end of *fangsung* ("relax and let go"). It is a sense of total relaxation brought about by "feeling" every sinew of the body coming to rest in natural repose while breathing out.

**Sun Si-Miao:** A Tang dynasty (AD 619–907) pioneering physician who established the first ever codes of practice in medicine.

***Sung:*** "To deeply relax." In tai chi, it is a deep sense of relaxation where the body moves or remains still, completely free from stress and tension; often seen written as *song*.

***Tai:*** "Grand/supreme." This tends to be used in the context of naming something that is held in high esteem and revered.

***Tai Chi:*** "Grand ultimate." The most common term for the health and martial art of tai chi chuan.

***Tai Chi Tu:*** "Yin and Yang symbol." This is internationally known as a symbol of balance and harmony.

***Tao:*** "The Way." In energy terms, the origin of everything in the universe.

**Taoism:** "The study of The Way." Along with Buddhism and Confucianism, these are the three main ancient branches of Chinese religion.

**Taoist:** "Follower of The Way." An orthodox Taoist would be someone who retreats from society, usually to a mountain retreat, in search of Enlightenment.

***Teh:*** "Character." A person's individual traits, their unique character, what makes them the person they are.

***Tien:*** "Heaven." In Taoism, *tien* refers to the sky and beyond, into the mysterious universe.

***Wai:*** "External." This refers to the outside of the body and the outside space through which the body receives its nourishment (*qi*).

***Wai Dan:*** "External elixir." *Qi* is absorbed externally, usually through qigong/*daoyin*, via the limbs (especially the arms), then guided inward to nourish the body.

***Wei Qi:*** "Guardian energy field." A protective field of energy that shields the body against "external evils," such as colds, influenza, and various other diseases.

***Wuji:*** "No extremity." This is when an internal condition prevails to merge Yin and Yang into one in perfect stillness.

**Wuwei:** "To do by non-doing." In the same way as it is said "Less is more" and "Anything forced cannot be sustained," it is best to swim with the current than against it.

**Xi:** "Breathing." This is primordial breathing in its purest sense, also known as "embryonic breathing."

**Xian:** "An immortal." The name given to a highly evolved human who has attained The Way.

**Xiao Zhou Tien:** "Small Heavenly Cycle." A microcosmic orbit of circulating *qi* that runs up the spine (*du*) and down the front of the body (*ren*) designed to keep the Yin and Yang of the body in equilibrium.

**Yang:** "The positive energy of The Tao prevailing throughout the universe."

**Yangsheng:** "Vitality, health, and longevity." This is another way to describe the Chinese art of living.

**Yaojing:** "Shaking energy." Used originally in Chinese martial arts but has now broadened to be used in releasing trapped *qi* through the whole body or zoned body shaking.

**Yin:** "The negative energy of The Tao."

**Yin Tang:** "Sky Eye point." Located centrally on the forehead and also known as "the third eye." Adepts train themselves to look through the Sky Eye with their minds in order to gain insights about higher planes of existence.

**Yong Chuan:** "Bubbling well." Known more commonly as Kidney 1, these acupuncture points are located on the centre of the balls of the feet. They are regarded as the location where the gravitational centreline of the body connects to the earth.

**Zhan:** "To stand." It refers to standing still like a post driven into the ground to create stability and "rooting" for body and mind.

**Zhang:** "Long." A word that takes on a much richer meaning when viewed through the minds of the ancient Chinese masters, compared with our modern interpretation.

**Zhen:** "Real." Used to define something that is real as opposed to assumed.

**Zhong:** "Middle/centre."

# Bibliography

Blofeld, John. *Taoism: The Quest for Immortality*. London: Unwin Paperbacks, 1986.

Cleary, Thomas. *The Essential Tao: An Initiation into Taoism*. San Francisco, CA: HarperCollins, 1993.

———.*Vitality, Energy, Spirit: A Taoist Sourcebook*. Boulder, CO: Shambhala Publications, Inc., 2009.

Cohen, Kenneth S. *The Way of Qigong*. New York: Ballantine, 1997.

*I Ching: Book of Changes*. Translated by James Legge. London: Constable and Company, Ltd., 1963.

Jwing-Ming, Yang. *Qigong Meditation: Embryonic Breathing*. 2nd ed. Wolfeboro, NH: YMAA Publication Centre, Inc., 2022.

Kaptchuk, Ted J. *Chinese Medicine*. London: Rider, 2000.

Lau, D. C. *Lao-Tzu: Tao Te Ching*. Reprint ed. London: Penguin Classics, 1964.

Newton, Peter. *Tai Chi and Qigong: The Ultimate Beginner's Guide*. Conwy, Wales: China Bridge Publications, 2000.

Tsung Hwa, Jou. *The Tao of Meditation*. New York: Tai Chi Foundation, Inc., 1983.

Veith, Ilza. *The Yellow Emperor's Classic of Internal Medicine*. Rev. ed. Boulder, CO: Shambhala Publications, 1995.

Windridge, Charles. *Tong Sing: The Chinese Book of Wisdom*. Edited by Cheng Kam Fong. London: Kyle Books/Hachette UK, 2018.

Winnicott, D.W. *Playing and Reality*. London: Routledge, 1991.

Wong, Eva. *The Tao of Health, Longevity, and Immortality*. Boulder, CO: Shambhala Publications Inc., 2000.

# Illustration Credits

## Earth Path—Introduction

**Figure 1:** Original *Daoyin Tu* silk painting. Artist: *Daoyin Tu*, a chart for leading and guiding people in exercise for improving health and treatment of pain containing animal postures such as Bear Walk. Origin: The images originally come from a Guiding and Pulling Chart excavated from the Mawangdui Tomb 3 (sealed in 168 bc) in the former kingdom of Changsha. Source: Wellcome Collection. Attribution 4.0 International (CC BY 4.0). www.wellcomecollection.org/works/sybqrqu7.

**Figure 1a:** Enhanced *Daoyin Tu* silk painting of Figure 1. This is a reconstruction of a Guiding and Pulling Chart excavated from the Mawangdui Tomb 3 (sealed in 168 bc) in the former kingdom of Changsha. Origin: The original is in the Hunan Provincial Museum, Changsha, China. Source: Wellcome Library, London L0036007. Wellcome Collection. Attribution 4.0 International (CC BY 4.0). www.wellcomecollection.org/works/rrb7c7cm.

**Figure 2:** 14th-century painting of Zhong-Li Quan instructing Lu Dongbin. Artist: Atelier of Zhu Haogu. Public domain. Wikimedia. www.commons.wikimedia.org/wiki/File:Zhu_Haogu%27s_atelier._Zhongli_Quan_Instructing_Lu_Dongbin._completed_by_1358._Chunyangdian,_Yonlegong,_Shanxi_Province.jpg.

**Figure 3:** Shao Yuan Jie, Zhengyi Dao's Taoist priest of mid-Ming Dynasty. Artist: 顧鼎臣撰—《賜號太和先生相贊》Public domain. Creative Commons—Public Domain Mark 1.0. www.commons.wikimedia.org/w/index.php?curid=79668198. Note: This is the acknowledgement to the provider of the Taoist priest image Shao Yuan Jie.

## Step 1

**Page 37:** AI generated using Adobe Firefly with the prompt "light shining through forest grayscale."

**Figure 8:** Elderly couple in red triangle crossing the road. Courtesy of https://pixabay.com/vectors/sign-old-people-crossing-elderly-24343/ (Free use download).

**Figure 9:** Positive old people image on road sign. Source: The Centre for Aging Better—Range of Free to Use Positive Icons. www.ageing-better.org. uk/news/dancing-couple-design-wins-age-positive-icon-competition

## Step 3

**Figure 17:** White Crane badge of office (rank), Qing Dynasty (AD 1644–1911). Public domain. Source: The Metropolitan Museum of Art. Courtesy of https://picryl.com/media/insignia-medallion-030dec

**Figure 18:** Crane with Bamboo (right of a triptych of White-Robed Kannon and Cranes). Artist: Japanese 17th-century artist. Public domain. Source: Minneapolis Institute of Art/Kano Tan'yu. www.collections. artmia.org/art/122117/crane-with-bamboo-attributed-to-kano-tanyu

**Figure 19:** *White Crane Airs Its Wings*. Image by wirestock on Freepik. www.freepik.com/free-photo/black-necked-crane-landing-ground-covered-snow_11890149.htm#from_view=detail_alsolike

**Figure 21:** Landing cranes. Image by wirestock on Freepik. www.freepik. com/free-photo/selective-focus-shot-three-red-crownedcranes-flapping-their-wings-kushiro-national-park_11526522.htm#query=White%20 Cranes&position=29&from_view=search&track=ais"

## Step 4

**Figure 27:** Shou Lao painted porcelain statue with peach and gourd. Artist: Qing Dynasty (18th century). Public domain. Source: Metropolitan Museum of Art. www.metmuseum.org/art/collection/search/47916

**Figure 28:** Emperor Huang Di. Public domain. Source: Wikimedia. www.commons.wikimedia.org/w/index.php?curid=48048

**Figure 29:** Lao Tzu. Artist: Unknown. 歷代名臣像解. Public domain. Source: Wikimedia. www.commons.wikimedia.org/w/index. php?curid=117214485

**Figure 30:** Tao Te Ching, 2nd century BC manuscript. Public domain. Source: Wikimedia. www.uploAD.wikimedia.org/wikipedia/commons/e/ed/Mawangdui_LaoTsu_Ms2.JPG

**Figure 31:** Chang San Feng. www.commons.wikimedia.org/wiki/File:Changsanfeng.jpg#/media/File:Changsanfeng.jpg

**Figure 32:** Li Ching Yuen. Public domain. Source: Wikipedia. www.en.wikipedia.org/wiki/Li_Ching-Yuen

## Step 7

**Figure 47:** The Spirit of a Still Heron © Tim Wilson / Unsplash. https://unsplash.com/photos/grey-heron-on-brown-wooden-dock-during-daytime-uUJOmCkhuZM

## Step 8

**Page 172:** tree image © Jeremy Bishop / Unsplash. https://unsplash.com/photos/sun-light-passing-through-green-leafed-tree-EwKXn5CapA4

## Final Comment

**Figure 49:** *The Daoist Immortal Lu Dongbin Crossing Lake Dongting.* Public domain. Source: Wikimedia Commons. Boston Museum of Fine Arts. www.commons.wikimedia.org Search: The Daoist immortal Lu Dongbin crossing Lake Dongting.jpeg

# Acknowledgements

I would like to sincerely thank my close friend Steve Morris for his excellent photography input. Steve has contributed most of the photographic images shown in the book.

I would similarly like to thank Stephen Croman who, despite having to contend with his personal health issues, has kindly contributed some supplementary photographs.

Thank you to Robert Awood of Cardrews Media, who helped me with the images for the book.

I am also grateful to Sabine Weeke and her team at Findhorn Press for believing in the potential of my work, and all the Inner Traditions team in the US who have helped make this book a reality. Thanks especially to my editor, Nicky Leach, for her patience, guidance, and kind words of encouragement.

Many thanks, too, to my incredible wife, Lesley, who initially thought *Oh, no, not again!* when I announced that I was writing my next book, but since then, has done nothing but support me throughout all the highs and lows of giving birth to a manuscript.

This is also an opportunity to thank my adult children, Richard and Janine (and son-in-law Pat), who are always there for me—not forgetting my precious grandson Arthur, who I hope will also benefit from the knowledge contained within the pages of this work throughout what I hope will be a long and healthy life.

# About the Author

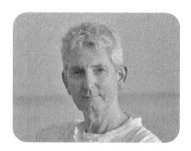

**Sifu Peter Newton** has spent more than 40 years researching and training in the ancient Chinese arts of tai chi chuan and qigong. In 1998, he made the bold decision to become a full-time professional instructor after a long career in construction management. The timing proved to be opportune as the demand for tai chi instructors outweighed the supply.

Peter was trained in a traditional way by three masters—Chu King Hung, Michael Tse, and Dr. Yang, Jwing-Ming—and has retained the principle of tradition in his current teaching. However, over the years, he has acquired the ability to adapt the science of these traditional Chinese arts to suit a variety of his clients, including international soccer players, major business clients, Parkinson's UK, MS Society, The Stroke Association, Kick-Start Cardiac Rehabilitation, MIND Mental Health Charity, Leonard Cheshire Acquired Brain Injury Unit, and North Wales Police Service.

Since his neck injury in 2007, Peter has dedicated all his time to promoting "medical tai chi," and he is now regarded as a pioneer in this field. Now, at the tender age of 68, Peter is more in demand than ever for his wisdom and teaching style. It seems the older he gets, the more people are attracted to what he has to say. For further support and advice please visit www.chinabridgetaichi.com

# Index